A Life Worth Saving

A Life Worth Saving

A Nurse's Journey from Sickness to Healing

ATIYA ABDELMALIK, PhD

XULON PRESS

Xulon Press
2301 Lucien Way #415
Maitland, FL 32751
407.339.4217
www.xulonpress.com

Edited by Xulon Press.

Printed in the United States of America.

ISBN-13: 978-1-6305-0694-0

*For Keemy and Mom: your love and light taught me
what it means to believe we're all worth saving!*

Table of Contents

Introduction ix

Part I: My Life 1

Buddy 3

Save Him 10

Finding Nemo 13

Just Keep Swimming 16

Made of Love 18

Little Atiya 20

Earth Family 22

The Window 28

Bad Food Love Affair 32

Ginseng, Tofu, and Monkey Bars 34

Nothing Stays the Same 37

As the World Turns 39

Family Ties 41

Farm School 43

I'm Not a Nurse 50

Denied 57

Why Me? 62

She's Alive 66

Triumph 68

These Four Things 75

A Broken Heart Still Beats 81

For Better or Worse 87

If Sorrow Comes Tomorrow 89

Forgiveness is Freedom 93

Part II: The Lessons.. **97**

   Lesson 1: The Journey is Not A Straight Line 99

   Lesson 2: What's Love Got to Do with It? Everything 102

   Lesson 3: Build-A-Body 106

   Lesson 4: Everyone Needs a Karen 112

   Lesson 5: Slow Down and Breathe.......................... 117

   Lesson 6: It's Not Worth the Pain........................... 121

   Lesson 7: Eviction Notices 123

   Lesson 8: Be Afraid of the Dark 125

   Lesson 9: Make Every Moment Count 131

   Lesson 10: The Voice Within.............................. 139

Part III: Why You Were Born **143**

   Atiya's Living Room 145

   If You Could Save One Person 149

   Not for You Alone 152

Epilogue.. **155**

Acknowledgments **159**

Introduction

YOUR LIFE IS A JOURNEY, A STORY CONSISTING OF CHAPTERS that bring you complete and utter joy and others that pierce permanent thorns in your side. As a child, I didn't have a clue as to the devastation my life would endure. When your nickname is Sunshine it is hard to believe that life really isn't a fairytale. Life—*real* life—can be both interrupted and disrupted. It hits all of us at some point in our lives, and for some of us, we don't have to wait until we're older to experience both life's beauty and brutality.

I started on the path of writing to help someone else overcome their giants, or so I thought. It all began with one woman who stood before me with tears falling down her round face. Her arms were stretched out when she grabbed my hands and asked for more. I had just finished speaking, sharing my story. She proceeded to ask me a question that has directed my path for more than ten years. She convicted me that day and I wanted to give her the more she asked for, a book to be exact. She needed something tangible to take home and, when needed, to open up a page and see the possibility in saving her life. Little did I know, the one who needed inspiring more than ever was the person who was asked to write the story—me. Every time I overcame a hardship, I'd put it in my survivor's manual, my book of lessons. Just when I thought the manual was full, that I've learned enough, loss and tragedy continued to find its way back to greet me. The tragedy that hit like a head-on collision not only knocked the wind out of my sails, but also annihilated my desire to live. It was an experience, a trauma that left me in a space of questioning my very existence. Giving up was a daily thought but something in my spirit wouldn't let me die. Surviving was coded in my DNA. My only option was to get up and keep moving forward. I was not going to allow physical, emotional, and spiritual decay to consume me from the inside out. I was going to survive to tell the story, survive to write new chapters. Survive until I could thrive. And, to give that woman something that would encourage her to do the same.

The lessons and the indomitable resilience of the human spirit have taught me how to move through the worst of life's pain while not forgetting the beauty in its triumphs. Abandonment, teenage pregnancy, abuse, disease, and more have all played a part in shaping who I am today. I must accept all parts of my journey, all parts of me.

In the deepest part of my being, I knew that my journey was not for me alone.

A Life Worth Saving is my story. My declaration and promise that no matter what, I would never give up. My journey is written in three parts. Part I is the story of my joy-filled childhood and the traumatic disruption of my family. It begins with my mom, Karima. A young, single mom of three children, my mom was my personal griot, history-sharer, and storyteller. She taught me the most valuable life lessons through her interesting and quirky way of teaching.

Part II contains lessons that will have you laughing in tears, nodding your head in agreement, and revealing your own epiphanies. I share these funny and sometimes painful lessons with hope that you will learn from the crooked paths of others—in this case, me. Letting go of the experiences that hold you captive. Letting go of the stories that no longer fuel who you desire to be. I share some of the lessons my mom taught me and some of the hard ones I had to learn for myself. How can my life and my lessons inspire you to cultivate a life that doesn't bow down to hardships? How do you forgive the unforgivable? How do you forgive yourself? How do you create new rituals of living so that you cherish people and experiences instead of things? How do you cultivate a practice of self-love? And how do you create a joy-filled life that's not determined by the storm you're passing through?

Part III, the final section of the book, is full of gentle nuggets; revelations that have helped me awaken to a life worth saving. There were several divine encounters that reaffirmed that my place and time on earth was for a much bigger purpose than just getting by and saving my own life. I truly believe that your world doesn't have to be turned upside down to know and do what's best for your life. Sometimes we get this worthy thing twisted. No matter what, you deserve to care for yourself, mind, body, and spirit like nobody's business. You deserve to live in a healthy vessel, one designed to take you to your purpose. The goodness of life and the painful but necessary growth experiences are yours to use for your own transformation. I'm doing just that and have shared my journey with the hope you'll do the same.

I came to discover what the prophet Jeremiah described as the Lord's promise of peace: health, healing, and the abundance of truth. That is what I want for you: to not only believe without a shadow of a doubt that your life is worth saving but also to go about the business of saving it. There are so many movements to follow. I hope you create your own. Sometimes this living at a higher energy is a tall order but I believe there's nothing more important than honoring your life, the most incredible gift you've been given. For when your vessel is full and overflowing you can pour into others, and when they walk up to you asking for more you'll be ready and equipped.

Part I

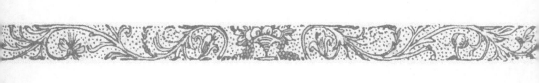

My Life

Buddy

SEEING DR. HANLON WAS THE FIRST STEP AFTER BURYING my son. Getting a dog was the second.

"Dogs are great for healing," Dr. Hanlon said. She shared so many ways to help me cope, by taking one step at a time. It was only two weeks earlier that I experienced the most unimaginable loss. I buried my oldest son, Hakeem, affectionately known as Keemy, and I was having a hard time trying to figure out how I was going to go on breathing.

I was one of the last to leave work that evening. I called my youngest son, Diante, and asked him to do research on where I could buy a puppy. I gave him a list of what I wanted in my first dog: preferably female, and a lap dog—also known as a pocketbook dog—was a must.

I was a little shocked when my son responded, "Mom, why don't you adopt a dog from a shelter?"

It was moments like these that made me happy my teenage son was thinking about helping others, including animals that were less fortunate. I thought it was a brilliant idea, but I told him that I wasn't too confident that my dream dog would be found in a shelter. In most of my encounters with animal rescues, I only found large dog breeds that couldn't possibly fit on my lap—and certainly not in my pocketbook.

"Mom, just go check it out. You never know," Diante insisted.

Tim gave me one of those looks that expressed he was not on board with my explanation as to why adopting a dog was a good idea. It was because of Dr. Hanlon's suggestion that I begged Tim to open our home to a dog. Yes, he thought seeing Dr. Hanlon was what I needed, but the dog suggestion was surely not on his approved list for coping mechanisms. I didn't know how Tim was processing what we were now experiencing. I'm sure that at our wedding three months prior, the thought that he would have to witness his wife move through such a devastating loss wasn't something that he, like any husband, had been preparing for. When I got in the car and told him I wanted to stop at the Humane Society, his reaction was far from approving. I shared with Tim the conversation I had with Dr. Hanlon. I was pulling out all the muscle I could use to convince Tim that this was a good idea. I even tried to use my nursing background to point out how service dogs visit nursing homes and hospitals and how horses are used in equine therapy. I wanted so much for him to understand that there was a method to my madness. A part of me didn't care about case studies or statistics demonstrating the healing power of animals. I wanted Tim to understand that this is what I *needed*. He tried his best to explain that we weren't ready for a dog.

"You're a cat person. You don't know a thing about caring for a dog. And who is going to care for it? What are you going to do while you're at work all day?" Tim asked.

They were logical and relevant questions, but he was asking them at the most illogical time in my life. I couldn't think that far in advance. I was trying to figure out my next breath and he was asking me to wrap my head around the next day.

"Please, let's just go and see. They probably won't have a small dog anyway," I replied.

Like in everything else, Tim knew he didn't have a chance. He explained that he understood, but he didn't envision a shelter dog in my future. Tim shared the same initial thoughts I had about going to a breeder and choosing my perfect pocketbook puppy.

"You know the shelter isn't going to have the dog you want," he said, still trying to convince me.

I didn't tell Tim I'd shared those exact thoughts with Diante. I didn't want to give him the satisfaction or any room to reinforce my doubts. I *needed* a dog.

I needed something I could cuddle and cry with. I needed something that I didn't have to explain my feelings or outbursts to, and something that would unconditionally lay by my side while I moved through the moments that rushed over me like huge waves, almost drowning me. I didn't need Tim's permission; I needed to inhale enough air to survive until the next tidal wave. But I wanted his understanding, his support, and a glimpse of faith that this would be good for me, and for the both of us.

It was December and already dark and cold outside when we left the office. I was filled with so many different emotions. I thought it was a slim chance that I would find the dog that met all my requirements. Although I believed a new addition to our family would be a vessel of healing, I was secretly afraid that attaching myself to something that would eventually die would add another devastation to my life.

We ended up at the Humane Society, which was five minutes away from my job.

Upon entering the shelter, I explained that I was there to see the dogs. Tim just stood there in silent protest. I knew he wasn't on board, but I couldn't focus on his needs. I was in a daze. Nothing seemed real to me. Moment to moment, my focus was on how I was going to survive this journey. I didn't have the capacity to process how adopting a dog would impact our lives. We would figure it out, one step at a time.

Warmth enveloped me as Tim and I headed to the entrance of the doggy quarters. This feeling was a sign that what I needed was waiting on the other side of the double doors. My furry companion would find a home, and I would find a way to move forward.

I so wanted Tim's attitude toward this step in the healing process to be different. I wasn't in a corner, numb and sucking my thumb. I was actively seeking ways to live despite my constant questioning as to why I was the one still breathing. I felt, for the first time, what it meant to be willing to lay down your life for someone else. I knew without a shadow of a doubt that I would have given up my life for my son to have another chance to live his. This deep and painful loss taught me in so many ways that *agape* love was real. Giving up my life in exchange for my son's life would not have required a second thought.

The odor coming from the dogs' quarters was overwhelming. I couldn't bring myself to look at Tim's face. We were dressed in our office best, and the stench was inescapable. If I had any chance of convincing Tim this was a good decision, the smell from the dogs' quarters cut that chance to zero. German shepherds, pit bulls, pit bull mixes, and other large dogs filled each crate. Some were barking while others pierced through your soul with their silent looks of despair.

It didn't look too good for me. I didn't see any cute, pocketbook dogs waiting to go home. But when we came to the puppy room, my heart began to race a little faster. This could be it. My anticipation was met with a cynical explanation from Tim that those cute little puppies were Labrador retrievers, and the "cute and little" would wear out in a few weeks.

"Atiya, you're looking at puppies that will grow to be seventy-plus pounds," Tim explained.

I was desperate, and in my moment of desperation, I was willing to overlook the paw size on those cute Lab pups. I convinced Tim to walk around just one more time. During this last trip, I stopped at every single kennel until I came upon one that contained three small dogs.

At first glance, they weren't aesthetically pleasing, but I was willing to mull over their descriptions hanging outside of the kennel. It was rather easy to eliminate two of the dogs, one of which was so ugly that thought of waking up to him would be a nightmare. I felt bad for feeling like this, but I needed comfort, and that face required something that I just didn't have to give.

I pointed out the last of the three to Tim. His name was Buddy, and he was a full-bred Yorkshire terrier.

"Tim, it's a Yorkie, just the dog I wanted," I said.

Tim looked at Buddy, then turned to me and said, "Atiya, there's no way that ugly, disheveled dog is coming home with us."

Tim had had enough and decided our trip to the Humane Society was over. I begged and pleaded that Buddy was the dog for me. All Buddy needed was a little love and a trip to the groomer. But Tim wasn't having it. His once silent protest was no longer silent.

I trailed behind Tim as he walked out of the kennel and through the double doors, leaving the stench and Buddy behind. I tried my best to beg with dignity, but it didn't work. I burst into tears. And not just quiet sobs of tears; no, these were tears of protest and heartache.

I don't know if Tim genuinely felt sorry for me, or if the embarrassment of his wife crying like a two-year old was too much to handle. After all, he would have looked like a total jerk if he continued to leave. After a few feet of trying to escape my cries, Tim turned around and asked for an adoption counselor. "My wife would like to see Buddy," he said.

The adoption counselor sent us into a room to wait for him to return with Buddy. He was indeed a Yorkshire terrier, but he was in bad shape. It was clear that Buddy wasn't taken care of. His teeth were rotted, his hair matted, and he was rather small, even for his breed.

Buddy sat on my lap with his face turned toward Tim. As the adoption counselor shared what history he knew about Buddy, Tim interrupted and asked where the horrible odor was coming from. It was Buddy's breath. Within a second, the adoption counselor leaned down and placed a bottle on the desk filled with a clear solution. He proceeded to tell us that Buddy's oral hygiene was less than stellar, but all we needed to do was place a few drops of the solution in Buddy's water bowl every day. *Check*, I thought.

Buddy let out a horrible cough and Tim asked, "What's wrong with the dog? Is he sick?"

The adoption counselor leaned down, placed a packet of pills on the table, and said, "Oh, dogs sometimes get a case of kennel cough. No need to worry. Just give him this medicine and it will clear right up." *Check.*

Tim asked, "Is there anything else you want to tell us about this dog?"

The adoption counselor replied, "Well, the dog is considered a senior dog—seven years or more. We don't know his exact age, but you get an adoption fee discount for that." *Check.*

This revelation was the first time in the process that I felt a hint of concern. I asked, "What's Buddy's life expectancy?" The last thing I wanted was to take Buddy home and end up burying him in a year.

The adoption counselor proceeded to share that small dogs usually lived much longer lives. Buddy, with proper care and nourishment, could live until the high-teens, which was a big deal in doggy years. I did the math and thought this could be all right, at least for me. But Tim still wasn't convinced. His last stand of protest was to explain how we didn't have any supplies at home, no food, no bowls, no leash, and no collar. Absolutely nothing. We were unprepared. The adoption counselor told us not to worry and made Buddy a care package containing everything we needed to get us through a few days. *Check.*

I walked out with a smile and dried tears plastered to my face. Tim's happiness was not yet evident and having to drive home with the windows down due to Buddy's unbearable breath didn't help our plight.

I made up "Buddy's Song" on our way home. It was a melody that went along with Sesame Street's "Elmo's Song." Buddy didn't care that I couldn't hold a tune, and that my singing voice could cause serious damage to human ears. Nope. My lack of singing ability didn't matter. I had Buddy, and Buddy had me. My heart began to beat again. It didn't take Buddy long to warm up. Our connection was instant. *Thanks, Dr. Hanlon*, I thought. I got my dog, and not just any dog, but a small pocketbook dog that knew his job was to show me love and for me to do the same for him.

As soon as I opened the door to our home, Buddy ran up the steps as if to say, "I'm home. Now which room is mine?" Buddy was well-behaved. Many people warned me about small dogs. Yappy and snippy, always ready to pounce, saying their bark is bigger than their bite. Not Buddy. He was pure, 100 percent sweetness. He was fully trained and even helped by training me. It was almost as if Buddy knew I was new to this. Despite having a horrible cough, some rotten teeth, and being in desperate need of a trip to the groomer, I witnessed from a little four-legged "buddy" what gratitude looked like.

On his first night in our home, I experienced a rough crying spell. Buddy made his way into my bedroom and, without having to do anything else, laid on my lap if to say, "I'm here, and you're not alone." As much as Tim would have liked to continue protesting, Buddy's heart was enough to melt Tim's reticence.

For the first time in weeks, I was showing proof of life. Buddy gave me something to care for, something to save. This little creature was dependent on me, and I on him. Buddy would look to me to provide him with the comfort of a loving home and the unconditional love he needed. He needed to not feel abandoned and alone in a shelter, and I needed something small enough to hold in my lap and stroke as the tears of pain fell down my face. I needed something that would travel alongside me on the long journey ahead. But it didn't last.

After having Buddy for forty-eight hours, I called the Humane Society and told them that Buddy was in severe respiratory distress. I found him earlier that morning in the back of my closet, balled up with wide eyes and struggling to breathe. This was the place Buddy was planning on taking his last breath. I knew the look. As a nurse, I had experienced that look that preceded death. I spent too many years being the one at the bedside holding a patient's hand as they transitioned. I was not accepting this, and made it clear to the Humane Society that they better save Buddy.

Save Him

THERE WAS NO WAY THAT AFTER BURYING MY SON, I WAS going to bury the pet that was going to help me through my journey of loss. This could not possibly be my reality. I couldn't wrap my head around what was happening. Tim and I were rushed into a small examination room at the veterinary hospital, waiting for *what's next*. In my heart and mind I knew I would lose him. The most hope-filled encounter I had in the past two weeks was being ripped away.

The veterinarian at the hospital reminded me more of a deer hunter than a vet. His large physique and bearded face looked out of a place in this setting. It was the look on his face that communicated what I had already known. I took a hard swallow and asked a question that was more like a statement: "There's nothing you can do for Buddy, is there?"

"I'm sorry. We should not have adopted Buddy out. Buddy didn't have kennel cough. He had severe congestive heart failure," said a staff member at the Humane Society.

"Are you kidding me?" I responded, heartbroken and angry.

The response confirmed this was not a joke. "No, we're very sorry. We're waiting on a volunteer driver to take Buddy to the emergency vet hospital to see if there's something they can do for him. We'll take care of the medical bills."

"I don't need anyone to take Buddy to the hospital. My husband and I will be there to get him," I said.

Tim was just as perplexed as I was. How in the world could this be happening? I tried to remain as calm as possible to help Buddy conserve

10

his energy. The "Buddy Song" was now painful to my own ears. A short drive felt like an eternity. The Humane Society notified the hospital staff that we would be arriving within minutes. It was clear the vet hospital got that message as Tim and I rushed through the doors to the wide-eyed vet technician waiting to receive Buddy in her outstretched arms. The veterinarian at the hospital was upset. More like angry. He couldn't believe the misdiagnosis.

I kept thinking back to when Tim asked the adoption counselor what was wrong with Buddy. We thought it was funny that every time Tim complained, the counselor leaned down from his chair and pulled out a remedy. Unfortunately, the pills for the kennel cough weren't the right cure for Buddy.

Tim stood on the periphery of the clinic room as I explained the life-changing events of the past few weeks to the vet. I needed Buddy more than anything, and Buddy needed me.

I was filled with a mix of emotions: Sad. Angry. Lost. My sharing didn't help the veterinarian deal with his own emotions; it only escalated the miserable place we both found ourselves. A place that surely didn't have a fairytale ending. Buddy would have to be put to sleep.

The veterinarian explained that although Buddy was from a small breed, the severe congestive heart failure caused his body to work too hard and contributed to muscle wasting, hence the reason for his size.

"Would you like to hold him during the process?" the veterinarian asked.

For the first time during this entire exchange, Tim spoke up, he said, "No, she doesn't want to hold Buddy while you put him to sleep." He looked quizzically, as if in his mind he was questioning, "Didn't you hear what she's already been through?"

I chimed in before my husband got totally out of character. "Yes, I'd like to hold Buddy."

You see, my son died alone. There was no one by his side. According to his medical records, my son was resuscitated eight times, and on the ninth they couldn't bring him back.

By the time I was notified, my son was already at the morgue. He died in a hospital room probably like the clinic room where we stood with the veterinarian. He died in a room filled with equipment, monitors, and strangers using advanced resuscitation methods to bring him back. He died, more than likely, without someone holding him, and helping him to transition with as much peace as possible. He died without someone telling him that he was loved, and that they were sorry they couldn't help him turn his life around. He died without me, his mother, by his side. His mother, the one who brought him into the world nineteen years, ten months, and three days prior to the day he died.

No, Buddy would transition differently. He would transition in my arms, wrapped in a blanket as I sang the "Buddy Song" to him. He would go out knowing that the last forty-eight hours of his life were filled with love, a home, and someone who truly thought the world of him.

"Tim, I'd like to hold Buddy," I said.

The veterinarian prepared me for every part of the process. He explained that Buddy's eyes would remain open even when he's gone, but that he would tell me when Buddy fully transitioned. He asked me if there was anything that I could focus on to make me feel just a little better. I said, "Yes, I'm sending Buddy to my son, Keemy."

Buddy was brought to me wrapped up in his blanket with a tiny IV catheter threaded and taped around his little paw. I held Buddy close. He looked up at me with those beautiful, big eyes. I sang the Buddy Song, and he loved it. I sang and cried as Buddy took his last breath in my arms.

I've never witnessed my husband question God. But, on this night in a small clinic room, with Buddy dying in my arms, and the veterinarian crying with me as he slowly pushed the substance that would relieve Buddy of his painful existence, my husband looked up and with an exasperated cry asked, "Why?"

Finding Nemo

THROUGHOUT THE INITIAL PERIOD AFTER MY SON'S DEATH, people with good intentions kept saying, "God doesn't put more on you than you can bear." I was going to scream if I heard that one more time. Whatever "strong" list I was on, I wanted off. Immediately.

Tim, a quiet and introspective person by design, went into a silent retreat. He knew there were no words or physical comfort to remedy the pain we were journeying through. In his eyes, I could see the trauma. Three months prior, he stepped out on faith and decided to love again after experiencing a painful divorce seven years earlier. I'm sure what we were experiencing together was not what he signed up for.

I remember listening to a sermon preached by Pastor TD Jakes on marriage. In his sermon, Pastor Jakes talked about choosing a mate that will truly support you and love you through the worst of times. When people get married, it is the most beautiful moment in time—for the most part. The day is filled with love and happiness. The real test of the vows committed on that day happens after you turn and face the sea of family and friends and embark upon your life together. And in just three short months, we knew the reality of "for better or worse." Tim was in shock. Newly married watching his wife suffer an unexplainable loss and the one thing that would provide emotional support, a dog, dies in her arms.

Tim went to work and shared what happened to Buddy. One of his staff members, an avid supporter of the Humane Society, took in the animals that couldn't find forever homes. It was amazing to find out that the ugly dog I had rejected before choosing Buddy ended up at her home.

Now she is what I call an angel, because that dog looked like it was part-ferret, part-cat, and part-animal that mankind hadn't discovered yet.

She called the Humane Society and set off a chain of events that put my life on a different path. She explained what happened with Buddy and asked them to fix this. Over the next month, I received phone calls from the Humane Society and had the first choice of the small dogs that came in for adoption. Each dog was supposed to be perfect for me, but my follow-up calls involved a Humane Society staff member telling me that the latest dog was "too old," "blind," or "just not the right one." Every time I got my hopes up there was always a reason why that dog wasn't for me. Growing up I never had a dog for a pet. I filled my time researching the emotional support a dog can provide. For me a dog would be my real-life Teddy Bear, soft and cuddly and providing the comfort I needed so desperately.

"We think we have the one for you," said a Humane Society staff member on the other end of the phone.

The dog's name was Enzo, and he was a six-month-old Morkie (a Yorkie and Maltese mix). Enzo's owner was a young professional who bought the puppy from a breeder but traveled too much for her job to adequately care for him. When she dropped him off, I was told tears streamed down her face when she had asked the staff to please find him a good home. The staff members told me that they had all turned toward one another and said, almost simultaneously, "Don't worry. We know exactly where Enzo is going."

Enzo had to be neutered, so I couldn't pick him up for another twenty-four hours. The Humane Society also decided that they were not going to house him in the kennel and would keep him in the executive director's office until I arrived. The staff knew what I had been through with Buddy, and they were doing their best to avoid any repeat heartache.

I tried not to get my hopes up too high, but my heart was racing and my cheeks hurt from smiling. I was going to get my pocketbook dog, and he was still a pup.

The day I arrived to pick up Enzo, I wore a brown, faux fur vest. I walked in and was escorted to the Executive Director's office. Enzo was a little shy and stayed in the arms of the staffer. The director's office was filled with all his belongings left by his previous owner. Saks bags were piled high with high-end food, treats, toys, handmade blankets, a dog carrier, and clothes.

The counselor reached down into a bag and said, "Yes, Enzo is definitely your dog," as he pulled out Enzo's brown vest with faux fur around the hood. Yes, Enzo was my dog.

I asked if Enzo was too old for me to change his name. The staff assured me that he wasn't too old. So, Enzo became Nemo. And, just like in the movie, the journey to finding him was filled with pain, love, and healing. Tim took me and Nemo back to his office. The employee, Margaret, that helped facilitate this entire process was there. Also, a professional photographer, Margaret captured our first picture together, the moment I felt my heart beat again.

Just Keep Swimming

TWO YEARS LATER, BECAUSE I BELIEVE ALL DOGS SHOULD have a companion, we adopted Dory, a Maltese, from Angels for Animals.

When we adopted Dory, she was extremely fragile and frightened. The rescue shared how Dory and the other dogs from a puppy mill were severely abused. Although Dory's long hair made it look as though she was in perfect health, she was merely skin and bones. My heart hurt. Tim, in his usual form, sat quietly as I filled out what felt like a hundred-page adoption document. He finally asked, "What do they want us to sign over? Our firstborn?"

Yes, it was that intense. Due to the abuse Dory experienced, the rescue wanted to ensure she was going to a home that would be able to manage the issues that come with a dog that has experienced such trauma. We were given a two-week trial period with explicit instructions that if Dory didn't work out, we could return her to the rescue. Dory's big eyes were lifeless. It was as if a lobotomy had been performed on her. She walked around zombie-like and crouched close to the ground when you came near. It broke my heart to watch Dory tremble in fear of any movement. Clearly, her experience with a raised hand meant a painful blow to her defenseless body.

Nemo's excitement for a new buddy quickly dissipated when his attempts to play with Dory were met with zero enthusiasm. She didn't walk upstairs, her tail didn't wag, and she walked in constant circles, a side effect from living in a cage. The foster parent described this behavior as "crate crazy."

Two weeks felt like two years. As a nurse, I had experienced first-hand the abuse against children. Instead of loving and protecting them, pain was inflicted. Many of these young patients required extensive therapy and other forms of restorative care to facilitate the healing process. I was experiencing these atrocities again, this time with a dog.

When the adoption trial came to an end, Tim and I were faced with the ultimate decision. Not much progress had been made in two weeks. Although Angels for Animals embedded a trial period, we knew there was no way we could return Dory. Poor Tim. He not only had to deal with me and my cyclical grief, but also a traumatized dog he too had to love back to life.

Dory has come a long way, thus proving a universal truth: love is a powerful healer. Nemo became her guide, her sidekick. You will never see one without the other. Dory, although considered a senior dog, plays, wags her tail, and bounces around in pure joy.

Tim and I are convinced that she doesn't quite have it all. He often teases and says there's a bag of nails in her head. I'm convinced there's only love inside. Dory and Nemo are eerily similar in personality to the fish characters from the movie, *Finding Nemo*. Yes, Dory is a special one, but when my days are low and I'm not feeling courageous, I hear Dory through her big, wide eyes telling me to just keep swimming!

Made of Love

ADOPTING MY DOGS WAS A LIFE-CHANGING EXPERIENCE.
The reasoning behind Dr. Hanlon's suggestion to get a dog is so clear to
me now. I'm convinced that these little creatures were created with 100
percent love. It's no wonder dogs are used to help people who are living
life differently-abled. Their presence can light up a nursing home and
with just a stroke of their fur, hearts begin to melt and smiles spread
across faces that only moments before lay empty from loneliness.

In a *New York Times* article, "The Healing Power of Dogs," the jour-
nalist shared anecdotal stories and research on the health and healing
power of dogs. In one study, it was demonstrated that pet owners
reported thirty percent fewer visits to the doctor and lower cholesterol
and blood pressure levels.

Crisis Center North, a local organization in Pittsburgh, has Penny,
the four-legged therapist. Penny takes her work seriously and partners
with human therapists to help facilitate the healing process for families
who have experienced domestic violence. She serves as a court advocate
and appears in court with her clients, bringing peace and security in the
most difficult circumstances. Penny is on a mission to heal the most
wounded of hearts and is a source of strength and comfort for victims.
A rescue herself, Penny is proof that healing comes in many forms.

As author Alexandra Horowitz describes in her book, *Inside of a
Dog: What Dogs See, Smell, and Know*, dogs can detect our health, our
truthfulness, our routines, and our stress levels. They are anthropologists,
studying, learning, and never getting out of touch with their human
companions.

As a nurse, I understand the importance of gathering evidence to prove a theory. But as a human being who has walked through traumatic experiences, I stand as a witness to the healing power of these creatures.

Tim underscores the healing Nemo and Dory have brought to our lives. Although there's a hint of jealousy, we have learned to co-exist. Nemo and Tim battle for my attention, and the love-hate relationship is cute to watch. When they play fight, Tim knows I only have one rule: let my little eight-pound ball of fur win. After all, he's made up of love.

I've learned a lot of lessons on this journey. One of the most important is the power of love. In the end, I believe love always wins.

Little Atiya

ANIMALS AND NATURE GAVE ME LIFE. EVER SINCE I WAS A little girl, my fascination with creatures fueled my desire to become a veterinarian. For as long as I could remember, my life was centered on caring for animals that knew no other way to exist but by loving unconditionally.

But my mom didn't like pets, and my heightened love for animals was met with much resistance. In my mom's eyes, cats and other animals were nasty creatures that jumped on furniture and ate off countertops. She merely tolerated my pets. Deep down I know my mom witnessed the joy I felt when I was out saving my neighborhood furry friends. As a child, it bothered me that stray animals were subject to the harsh realities of winter. I often took the liberty of turning our apartment building's utility closet into a rent-free pet rescue. During the brutal winter months, I would go on a quest to find stray cats and bring them there to live. Before having to say goodnight, I spent as much time as I could with them playing on the second-floor landing of our building. I could hardly sleep, anxiously waiting to check up on them in the morning. But there were unfortunate and sad mornings when I opened the doors of the utility closet only to find that my TLC wasn't enough to save my rescues from the harsh winters.

For a long time, caring for strays and classroom pets was as close as I got to having my own. I enjoyed picking up insects and placing them in jars, and it was easier sneaking these low-maintenance pets into our apartment. It's interesting how life changes you. I can remember loving insects and slimy creatures. Today, however, if I mistake a false eyelash

I removed for an insect, I go into a full-blown panic attack. Things that once were the epitome of my joy have now become a scene from a horror movie.

I'm telling you, it felt like Heaven opened when my mom finally gave up the fight to deprive me of pets. Sometimes I wonder if she gave in because she witnessed how happy I was around animals, or if it was her attempt at trying to get rid of the other creatures taking up residence in our apartment. You know, the small, grey ones with tails. It didn't matter what her reasoning was. All that mattered to me was that I was finally going to have a pet to call my own.

Ms. Rhoda, my first grade teacher at Powell Elementary School, was a blessing. She was the closest person to me that shared a deep love for animals. Her classroom was a living, breathing zoo. Ms. Rhoda gave me an outlet to love and care for the pets that lived in our classroom. She could always count on me to volunteer to take the pets home for the weekend. My mom was not happy when I showed up with a rabbit for the weekend, but for whatever reason I seemed to get my way. I learned all the regular school stuff you're supposed to as a first grader, but what captivated me the most was what I learned about animals. Rabbits, turtles, mice, and snakes were just a few of the creatures that shared our classroom space. I didn't think there was anything I couldn't like about animals—until I learned what snakes ate for breakfast.

The first time I had my heart broken was witnessing a poor little mouse have his life squeezed right out of him. The kids huddled around the snake aquarium and anxiously waited for Ms. Rhoda to drop the unsuspecting mouse into the snake's den. It was unbearable to hear my fellow first graders oohing and aweing in anticipation of the poor mouse's demise, and hard for my first grade mind to wrap itself around that revelation.

That was my first experience with trauma. I cried profusely upon watching the snake take delight in feeding time. Why couldn't the snake munch on greens like my family did?

Earth Family

WE DIDN'T EAT MEAT IN OUR HOME, AND WE WERE THRIVING. We didn't get sick, and when a sickness even threatened us, my mom was ready with the arsenal of herbs and natural remedies she bought from Chinatown and the Ecology Co-op.

My mom's forceful nature came in a small, but mighty package. I love listening to my Aunt Annie describe how tiny my mom was when she started walking at six months old. Hearing my mother described as feisty even as a baby was so in tune with how she lived her adult life.

Mom didn't follow the conventional way of thinking, believing, or living. Far from a conformist, my mother often chose the road less traveled. At the young age of sixteen, my mom converted to Islam and changed her name from Shirley to Karima. By the time she was eighteen years old, my mom had lost both parents. With just one sister and proceeds from an insurance policy that was blown in the wind, life was even more difficult.

She was a single mom raising my older sister, Samira, when she married my Abi. He was twenty years old and ran an import/export business in West Philadelphia. My parents weren't the typical couple. They were young, driven, socially conscious, Muslim, and vegetarians. They divorced when I was only two years old. Although my Abi was active in raising me, my early years were spent with my mom.

It was me, my mom, and my older sister, but it was no secret that my mom craved a son. Her blessing in the form of my brother, Yusef Moswen, came in 1977, five years after me. We called my brother by his middle name, Moswen. He was her light. The overwhelming love for her baby boy was further demonstrated by my mom's intent to breast-feed him until he was three years old. I swear he was at least four, but my mom never owned up to that timeline. As far as me and Samira were concerned, our little brother was way too big to be walking up to my mom, lifting her shirt, and standing under it breastfeeding. But, I'll give my mom this one and say the magic number was three years old.

I didn't realize until I was much older how young my mom was when she had us. Nothing she did was the norm for a teenage mother. Looking back, I have no idea how she cultivated such a healthy and eclectic lifestyle while carrying such a huge responsibility. By any means necessary, my mom was not going to allow single parenting, a fixed income, or a community that didn't share her values to dictate the type of life she was going to provide for her children.

My mom was mindful of our influences; there were no televisions in our apartment until we were much older. My mom was particular about television viewing and its power on a young mind. She believed that stimulation should come from reading, touching, and doing, instead of sitting and watching. Our days were filled with trips to the Please Touch Museum, The Franklin Institute, and The Afro-American Historical and Cultural Museum, destinations that became our regular stomping grounds.

We were nicknamed the "Earth Family," and everything about us made the name stick. There wasn't anything my mother couldn't do using available resources. If we didn't have an outfit to wear to school, my mom would whip out the sewing machine and make dresses for my sister and me. In thirty minutes flat, we were out the door looking like twins donning our homemade attire. Oh, and the shoes nailed our earth family status. You know, the comfortable earth shoes that are popular today? They were surely not runway-worthy back then (in all honesty, they are still not runway worthy). There was nothing glamorous about a brown, wide shoe with ridges that conformed to your feet. I guess they were the best choice when, like my mom, your feet served as your main source of transportation. I'll be honest; knowing better doesn't mean you do better because you won't catch me wearing those shoes today, no matter how good they are for my feet.

As the Earth Family, it was not unusual to see Karima and her three children walking everywhere. My mom owned only one car when we were younger, and it was a Volkswagen Karmann Ghia that could not possibly fit four people. It barely fit one. So, we walked everywhere or rode SEPTA, Philadelphia's transportation system. My mom, in her petite 4'11 frame, walked as if turbo jets were attached to the back of her shoes. Those little legs did so much in a day's travel, from bringing groceries home from the Ecology Co-op to taking us to the West River Drive to feed the ducks. I tried hard to mirror my mom's pace, but distractions surrounded me.

"Atiya, stop acting so spaced out and keep up!" I heard that almost every time I traveled with my mom on these trips.

Yes, you could say I was a little spaced out. In my mind, everywhere I traveled was an adventure. I made up all kinds of imaginary stories, including people that came with real-life personalities. It was my version of fun while we trekked around the city.

I think what my mom hated most about walking with me was my obsession with animals that didn't make the safe passage across the street. Since I wanted to be a veterinarian, these animals represented an opportunity to get a head start on performing autopsies.

"Atiya, get away from the dead cat. That's disgusting," my mom would say. I didn't think it was disgusting, but I wasn't planning on arguing with my mother, who wasn't fond of having to repeat things.

Fancy clothes, cute yet uncomfortable shoes, and food I was forbidden to eat also fascinated me. I dreamt of a refrigerator, freezer, and cupboards lined with all things in a box. Cereal, ice cream, candy, soda, and meat would have helped me fit in with the rest of the neighborhood. When it comes to food, Philadelphia is known for cheesesteaks, Italian water ice, Tastycakes, and soft pretzels. My mom would not entertain us having so much as one bite of those foods. Eating refined sugars and all the things kids loved were out of the question. If we wanted soft pretzels, my mom would make them from scratch using whole-wheat flour, but a cheesesteak? Don't even think about it.

Although we had cupboards in our kitchen and a refrigerator with a freezer, there was never any food in them, at least nothing that lasted more than a few days. If you searched you would only find herbs, ginseng, and good old Golden Seal. My mom believed that anything that could last for months or even years was not something she wanted in our bodies. My mom walked to the co-op every two to three days to make sure we had fresh fruit and vegetables. Yes, we belonged to the clean plate club, but it was a plate with proper portion sizes, wholesome food, and no second servings.

The Earth Family way of life was exactly that: our way of life. Although I felt like I was missing something, I enjoyed every meal my mother prepared for us. I felt safest eating this way inside our apartment where this way of life was normal.

Weekend trips to my Abi's house didn't give me a chance to indulge because both parents drank from the Earth Family fountain. Our water didn't even come from the store. My mom and her sister, Aunt Yakini, would pack us up early on Saturday mornings to take a trip to Chester County, a suburb outside of Philadelphia, to draw our water from a "real" spring—yes, they existed. What felt like a road trip across a few states just to get water was only an hour's drive from home. We were there to help, but admittedly, my siblings and I did more playing and getting wet than filling up gallon jugs of water. At home, we neatly lined up the water bottles alongside the kitchen wall. As each jug was emptied, we would prepare to start the process all over again.

Leaving our urban dwelling to travel to the spring was an adventure. As a child, I would tell people we were going away on a long trip. Calculating distance and understanding directions was not my strong suit. It's still not, so when Tim starts talking about, "Well, if the sun rises in the east..." I give him the side-eye and request the "directions for dummies" answer.

Our vegetarian lifestyle wasn't a great way to make friends either. Some of the most hurtful memories from my childhood were the teasing from kids. I coveted their fancy, tin lunch boxes with cartoon characters. Inside was filled with candy, Hoagies, chips, and drinks that came in a cool barrel replica known as HUGS.

My mom, on the other hand, sent us to school with homemade brown paper bag lunches packed with banana and honey sandwiches, and on other days bean sprout and tofu on whole grain bread. My mom never fell short in the lunch creativity department. I'm sure the whole grain bread my mother bought came straight from the farm to our table. The bread was super dark, and it looked like they just glued grains on top of it. My favorite was the tofu sandwich with bean sprouts and avocado. Sure, my lunches were pleasing to my young palette, but they weren't what everybody else ate. And for that, lunchtime became one of the most miserable periods of my day.

No matter how great my sandwiches tasted, I would rather be accepted than enjoy the nutritious meals my mother made for me. So, I learned how to deal with the food bullies by hiding in a stairwell during lunch period. The stairwell was my magical hiding place; it allowed me to escape the finger-pointing, yelling, and ugly faces when I opened my brown bag lunch. The stairwell protected me from questions like, "What's that?" "Is that real meat?" "Why is your bread so dark?" Lunchtime should have been a fun and happy experience, but I was always afraid of being discovered in my magical hiding place. Switching my eating location became an endless game of hide-and-seek.

They say when you know better, you do better, but at that young age, I didn't have a clue as to how good I had it. My food wasn't plastered on TV, enticing me to beg my mother to purchase it during her next trip to the grocery store. Tofu, avocados, and bean sprouts weren't on the top-ten list of foods kids asked for and being healthy wasn't televised or cool. It didn't fit into the food industry's plot to make money; they were more interested in leaving a devastating legacy of sickness. The kids at my school had all the name-brand, processed foods filling their lunchboxes. They could hold a contest about which white bread was the best: Wonder vs. Stroehmanns.

It wasn't cool being different and singled out. Thank goodness for my mom's circle of friends. She made sure we were around like-minded families. I was in a safe environment, where tofu was more common than chicken. Those times were the best because there was no reason to pretend I was something that I wasn't.

The Window

THE ECOLOGY CO-OP WAS A SMALL STOREFRONT THAT SAT at the corner of 36th and Powelton Avenue, in the heart of the University City neighborhood of West Philadelphia. Each section of the store was packed to the brim with everything my mom needed to whip up a healthy meal. The co-op reminded me of a glorified shack that welcomed people who had one goal in mind: nourishing their bodies with food from the earth. There was no Whole Foods or Trader Joe's back then. The co-op was it for us.

I savored the moments when my mom allowed me to accompany her on these Co-op trips. I wanted so badly to be with my mom, but my slow pace would turn a twenty-minute walk into a forty minute one. Quite frankly, trips alone were probably my mom's way of getting a much-needed break. I got anxious when my mom started preparing for her trip. She would grab her neatly folded brown paper bags from the bottom cabinets underneath the sink. Recycling wasn't cool or sexy back then, but my mom, like in most aspects of her life, was ahead of her time. I desperately desired to be in my mom's presence, even if it meant I would have to nearly run to keep up with her pace.

My big sister, Samira, was the designated babysitter. But instead of being a responsible one, she used my mom's departure as a great opportunity to practice her boxing skills on my pencil-like frame. Like many siblings, we fought. Now, when we reminisce about our childhood, we find ourselves focused on what irritated my sister the most: my overwhelming obsession to be with my mom and my early teen years in the makeup fast lane. The highlight of the early teen years was my decision to learn how to safely escape my sister's grasp by jumping out of my second-story bedroom window when I refused to wash the makeup off my face and she refused to allow me to walk out the door with it on. We laugh in hysterics today, but back then it wasn't funny. The window became a symbolic oxymoron. As a little girl, the window represented a prison that kept me from my mom, and as a teenager, it became my escape.

I get it now, but just like I couldn't understand why I had to eat food that was good for me, I didn't get my sister's version of protecting me.

Samira was quiet; she kept to herself and didn't bother anyone. But you could be certain that if you picked a fight with her, you would surely regret it. The only benefit of her Mike Tyson-like behavior was that she wouldn't allow anyone else to pick a fight with me.

There's beauty in getting older. In my case, I became taller than Samira and this added height gave me an advantage. Our last fight took place in our cramped apartment bathroom, and all it took was for me to take her knee and jam it up to her chin. I won by TKO, and this was our turning point. The right neurons started firing in her brain, and she finally realized that her baby sister wasn't the enemy. This final standoff was the beginning of a beautiful sisterhood that grew into the most rewarding friendship, one that is the strongest to this day.

No one believes these stories when they meet Samira. She is the most selfless, giving, and loving person. She has spent her entire adulthood caring for others, including me. She is the one that we all lean on (albeit, too much) and I can't imagine life without her. I get to have a bestie and sister in one, and it simply doesn't get much better than that. She's the kind of person I wish for everyone on a lifesaving journey. But I still wouldn't suggest testing her, because you never know when Mike Tyson might make a return appearance.

Before leaving for the Co-op, my mom would give her normal speech to prep my baby brother and me for her departure. I know Samira didn't like being left with us, but I don't think she had the same desire to hang on the back of my mother's swift feet to go grocery shopping.

"Atiya, I'll be right back. Do not hang out the window, screaming after me," my mom said.

My poor mom would have to go through the "trip-to-the-Co-op-routine" with me on way too many occasions. No matter how many times she repeated the words, "I'm coming right back," I'd still act like a complete nut and hang half my body outside our second-floor apartment window. I'd hang as far as I could without falling head-first, using my feet as an anchor while hollering for my mom to come back and get me. My mom was so embarrassed by my behavior. I'm sure my neighbors gave her the side-eye as she put on a smile pretending her daughter wasn't acting a fool. Despite several trips back to the apartment to try to get me to settle down, my mom finally had to give up, ignore my cries, and continue her trek to the Co-op. I wasn't fully aware and probably didn't care that my little brother picked up this bad habit of mine. When he was old enough, he joined me in what I now realize was the most ridiculous, spoiled brat routine.

Samira swore up and down that the cause of our obsession with our mom was due to breastfeeding. She would proudly state she was bottled-fed, hence the reason why she didn't behave the way we did. I don't know why I couldn't breathe without my mom; all I knew is that I wanted to be her shadow.

We called my mom "Ummi" from the time we could talk. *Ummi,* in the Swahili language, means mom. But I think the reason why I eventually stopped calling my mom Ummi was due to the incessant teasing from the kids in my neighborhood. I was teased for being different, I was teased because of the way I dressed, I was teased because of the food I ate, and I was teased for the endearing name I called my mom.

"Ummi, please take me with you," I would scream after her.

I didn't care that Samira would look at me with pure disgust. I wanted my mom, my Ummi. I never wanted to be without her, and although it was hard to keep up with her, I'd rather run with my little feet to keep the pace than wait for her to return.

The "can't-breathe-without-my-mom behavior" caused a lot of emotional pain for me as I got older. When our lives shifted and shattered, I began searching for love that could only come from my mom. And that search led me down a pain-filled road.

Bad Food Love Affair

THE TOUGHEST PART OF GROWING UP IN AN URBAN COMMU-
nity with so many families who lived different lifestyles was the daily
temptations. Children want so much to be accepted and to fit in with
everyone else. I was not an exception and accepting my mother's healthy
choices was a tall order.

Block parties were a popular pastime in my Philadelphia neighborhood. The city allowed residents to close the streets to traffic, play games
all day long, listen to loud music, and eat. Apart from not being able to
indulge in the forbidden foods, I loved attending block parties. I was
miserable not being able to eat the food, and dodging the temptation
was impossible.

Neighbors grilled hamburgers and hotdogs, drank HUGS, and ate
potato chips and candy. We were only allowed to play. These events
made me create an imaginary world. In my mind, a pear with its interesting shape became a chicken drumstick, and tofu on whole grain bread
was a lunchmeat sandwich.

My first attempt at defying my Earth Family lifestyle happened at a
block party during the heat of the summer. My mother warned us that
there would be no eating at our neighbor's home. I heard her, but I had
already made up my mind how I was going tear into a hotdog. What my
mom didn't know wouldn't hurt her, and the aroma of the fried hotdog
had lured me into its delicious trap of all things forbidden.

My sister Samira and I had a lot of friends in the neighborhood.
One neighbor lived in a small house on the corner of our block. They
were the Daniels, and their home was always full of life, music, and food.

We got along well with them. Although we were different in the way we lived, they accepted us. I don't think they ever went as far as to sample our food, but it didn't matter if we were friends. This was one family where we felt safe to be exactly who we were.

Their home was the perfect opportunity to eat meat, especially since we didn't have to worry about them snitching. I wanted all the fixings on my hotdog. My mouth watered in anticipation as I waited for the final preparations. This was a big deal. I was finally getting my chance. A brand-new bike couldn't have topped this experience. Once the hotdog was ready and handed to me on a crisp, white napkin, I raised it to my mouth and opened wide. Just as the hotdog was making its final landing, my mouth immediately shut, my eyes opened wide, and the joy was sucked right out of me.

The hotdog was so close to my lips that I could taste it, but seeing my mom's face as she approached me ended my first love affair with bad food. I don't know which I was sadder about: my mom finding out that I wanted to eat the same food as my friends, or the fact that I might not have another chance with a hotdog again. Karima—not Ummi—walked in, and the fairytale moment I'd been waiting for all my life turned into a nightmare. What was even more puzzling was my mom's timing. How was it humanly possible that she would walk in at the exact moment the hotdog was entering my mouth?

The scene didn't end well. The hotdog was in just as much trouble as I was. Its life ended in the trashcan, and I was marched out of the house with a phony smile plastered on my mom's face, a smile that meant I was in big trouble.

My mom couldn't understand why I would want to eat this crap. Despite her lectures about the benefits of our vegetarian, whole foods lifestyle, my young mind could not accept that I wasn't missing out by not eating like everyone else.

Ginseng, Tofu, and Monkey Bars

MY MOM DIDN'T USE SINGLE MOTHERHOOD AS AN EXCUSE to fill us with quick-fix, boxed foods. Instead, she engaged us in the preparation and cooking process after her trips to the Ecology Co-op.

If we wanted peas, taking them out of the pod was the only way we were going to get them. They were contained in their natural package and removed by our hands. If we wanted corn, we learned to remove it from the cob.

My mother's healthy lifestyle didn't end with what we ate. She deliberately exposed us to arts and culture. Meditation and yoga as much as we could do at our young age was a key component of our lives. There was a code my mother and her Earth Family friends followed, a code that my siblings and I couldn't appreciate: honor the earth, the fuel it produces, and the experiences that illuminate it.

During our trips to Chinatown, located in the downtown section of Philadelphia, I would imagine that we were in China. I imagined that the buildings, people, and food were just like they were in the real destination. If we were lucky, my mom would treat us to the Chinese restaurant that made tofu, brown rice, and vegetables. Our trips would end with my mom picking up a box of ginseng. The ginseng was packed in a nice row of small liquid vials. Every morning before going to school, I would open the box, remove one vial, and drink the liquid. I loved the taste, so my mother never got a protest out of me when it came time to have my daily dose.

I can't say the same for when I had to drink Golden Seal. If we showed the slightest sign of a bug, my mom would open the Golden

Seal capsules, mix the powder in water, and make us drink it down. The concoction had a terrible smell, and even worse, the taste was awful. If I was really sick, I got better quickly especially if there was a threat of having to drink Golden Seal. Even if I had to fake healing.

My mom refused vaccinations for as long as she could. I'm not sure if and when we finally received our shots, but I remember my mom in the school's office fighting to protect her children from getting who-knows-what injected into their bodies.

My mom's protests didn't end with school; family and friends got lectures or handwritten notes about what we could eat while visiting. I remember one holiday when visiting my paternal grandmother, whom I affectionately call "Nanny," I had to carry a note explaining what I could and could not eat. Most did not appreciate my mom's adamant approach to policing our nutritional plan. Some may have thought what I really needed was some meat on my bones.

I guess there was some truth to my small frame, since my godmother gave me the nickname "T-Bone." When I think back, I wasn't skinny; I was healthy. Our lives were filled with the same principles we're trying to deposit into families and communities today. Eat a healthy, balanced meal, engage in physical activity or play, find healthy ways to manage stress, and get connected with people. Yes, my mother was way ahead of her time, but on time, because the foundation she laid helped me return to a way of living that was most critical when my health was in crisis.

We didn't stay in the house watching television all day. As soon as we woke up, my brother and I would eat breakfast and go outside to play. Mud and snow were my favorite toys. It's probably hard for people who know me to believe that I once loved winter, but I did. Making snow angels was the best, and mud pies were an absolute delight. Give us pieces of sidewalk chalk and a clean pavement and it was turned into an oversized board game, hopscotch, four square, and kickball. The playground was right around the corner from our apartment building. Meeting up with friends to spend hours on the swings, sliding boards, and monkey bars filled my life with joy. It was simple, pure fun that fueled my childhood.

Nothing Stays the Same

MY MOTHER TRIED SO HARD TO MAINTAIN A HEALTHY LIFE-style for us, but things became increasingly difficult as we got older. When my mom landed her dream job as a radio personality at a popular station in Philly, her career opportunity became the crack in the door that allowed me to manipulate my way into a real-life Candyland game. Working overnight and weekends took its toll on my mother's schedule. I quickly found out that her lack of energy and daytime naps were the best times for me to ask for a quarter to play the arcade games. I was pretty sure my mother would not be popping up like she did at the block parties. No, I would finally be able to freely pop colorful Mike and Ikes and Now and Laters into my mouth.

There were moments that my mom would bend just a little and allow us to indulge in the occasional treat. One of our favorites was chewing gum, and our excitement over chewing gum was pathetic. Our desperation hit an all-time low when my siblings and I decided to save our gum in the butter compartment of the refrigerator. It was a grand idea until we couldn't remember which piece belonged to whom. After trying to come up with a logical approach to determine the rightful owner of the hard gum pieces we decided a simple game of "eeny, meeny, miny, moe" would do the trick. Yes, disgusting, but worth it. Chewing through the cold and hardened piece of gum was like trying to soften a rock. It's shocking we didn't break a tooth. Samira denies she was ever a part of our ridiculous plot to save the gum. I think my mom sometimes feeding us cashews from her mouth, calling us her baby birds, and sharing gum has scarred my sister to this day. My sister has such a phobia of the possibility of exchanging any fluids she won't even think about letting you drink out of the same cup or share a spoonful of anything with her.

My first taste of candy was everything I dreamt of, and the cherry, lime, banana, and lemon Now and Later flavors were the best. I learned that sugar is a drug, and the rush kept me going back for more. I was relentless in feeding the habit.

My mom must have thought I'd fallen in love with arcade games based on my daily twenty-five cents requests. I would run down the street from our apartment building and take a shortcut through a vacant lot on Haverford Avenue just to get to the forbidden treats. I wish I could say my deception stopped at candy. But by this point, I had a solid plan that worked every time: wait until my mom was either distracted or tired and bug the crap out of her for quarters.

Candy was a great first love, but it didn't fully satisfy my cravings. I knew I needed to devise a plan to get more money to graduate to the forbidden meat. I always envied my friends who would go to Larry's corner store and come out with the juiciest hamburger on a white bun with cheese, mustard, and ketchup. I thought if I could just get an additional quarter, I'd have enough for one cheeseburger. Well, it didn't take much to weasel my mother out of fifty cents. Even when she became suspicious, I crafted a story that would buy me time and get her off my scent.

Trips to my relatives' homes also gave me an excuse to wear my woe-is-me face, with lips poked out and belly protruding as if I was one of the kids on the *Feed the Children* television campaign. What my mother was doing was something few people could appreciate. She tried desperately to change the trajectory of our lives. She didn't allow our physical surroundings to dictate the life we would live. A food desert or living in the "hood" wasn't going to win, at least not while Karima was wide awake. I didn't honor this lifestyle or appreciate the great effort my mom put in to trying to live against the grain.

As the World Turns

WHERE YOU LIVE MAKES A DIFFERENCE. PLACE MATTERS. The newness of the apartment we moved into was great, but the community we moved from and the new development, although only separated by a few blocks, were two different worlds.

It's interesting how a few feet can drastically shift your existence. That's exactly what it did in our lives. It was as if an imaginary line was drawn. One side was filled with hope, the other with struggle and despair.

The apartment development was in a neighborhood filled with rowhomes. The beige, stucco, brown-trimmed buildings contained two apartments on three floors. The building we lived in was on a busy street sandwiched between two bars.

There were perks to moving. We lived within walking distance of the Philadelphia Zoo, the Art Museum, and my favorite place: The West River Drive, also the place along the river that I buried my beloved cat, Sapphire. My siblings and I developed new friendships and got to explore new sites, including the playground and the library. I never felt comfortable going to our neighborhood's community center. Kids had a streak of meanness; yes, bullying isn't something new. I was much more content with animals than people.

By the time I was in high school, I was eating anything, watching soap operas, and wearing makeup. Cheesesteaks, hoagies, soft pretzels, hotdogs, candy, and sugary cereals—nothing was off limits.

Our once family-oriented, working class neighborhood was under full assault. When the community started to deteriorate, drugs and death became a fixture in a place where I once found great joy. I begged my mom to move, but I didn't understand what moving entailed. In my mind, all we needed to do was pack up and find a new home. I couldn't process that it took more than a desire to move. It took money and resources, something that we had limited amounts of. These are the concepts in life that children are often shielded from. I couldn't wrap my head around why my mom wouldn't just leave the place that was destroying us. My mom did her best to explain, but, in my mind, I thought that if something was causing harm, you could just leave it behind.

The once vibrant space filled with children laughing and playing and working playground equipment became a dark and desolate place where you could find empty crack vials and paraphernalia. We weren't protected from the destruction. It wasn't an adult secret, hidden out of sight. It was as if we were meant to be witnesses to the end of our future. The adults may have been the targets, but the children were the casualties of this war.

No longer was it safe or fun to wake up and look forward to going outside to play. Homes that were once a refuge, a place to play, succumbed to abandonment. Hope: abandoned. Dreams: abandoned. Life: abandoned. Destroyed by small, but mighty, white "rocks."

A neighborhood of summertime block parties became a ghost town with empty swings and hoop-less basketball courts. Families were rendered inconsequential. A kryptonite was mass-produced and destroyed even the strongest of families. Crack was the Hiroshima, the Vietnam of my generation. As devastating as it was in first grade to witness a snake squeeze the life out of a mouse, that experience became a fairy tale memory in comparison to the annihilation I witnessed caused by a weapon called Crack.

Family Ties

At least when we fed the classroom pet snake, the mouse's destruction was swift. It swallowed the mouse whole, preventing a long, drawn-out process of suffering. But when the snake showed up in our family, it killed us slowly, although not softly. I'll never forget the night we were torn apart, literally from each other's arms. The three of us were in a circle, holding on for dear life. My Abi, aunt, and baby brother's dad were all there to whisk us into separate homes. They had said it was for the best. Our faces, our pain, our cries, told a different story.

We wanted so much to stay together. We wanted so much to be with our mom. She was my sunshine. No matter how dark it became, I knew she would come back. That night still wrestles me in my dreams.

We held on for as long as we could. The circle was broken by three adults trying to do what was right, but they didn't understand that separating us, three siblings, was the absolute worst thing they could have done. I never returned—at least not for good.

I stayed with my dad for a brief period, returning to my mom for small stints. It's interesting how the mind plays tricks on you. My sister Samira and I were the oldest, in our early teens, my brother, the youngest and most vulnerable, was the one who wasn't old enough to remember the good old days. It was in this moment that being called the Earth Family and hiding in the stairwell of my elementary school wasn't so bad after all. Samira remembers the series of events around our separation differently. I think it's all in our design. My mind has chosen to recall the timeline in a manner that reduces the heart trauma. What I know for sure is that I wanted to be with my mom until a chronologic period that prepared me for "real" adulthood. My heart was never granted its greatest desire.

There's a period in my life, a long one, which is so dark I believe I chose to permanently delete the memories only for them to creep their way into my sleep. Sleep, the most precious time when my cells should be about the healing process, they are instead being disrupted by painful memories of a time that aches for the light.

Farm School

MY CHILDHOOD LOVE AFFAIR WITH ANIMALS WASN'T JUST a phase. I'm sure my mom wished it would have been short-lived, but it intensified as I got older. My cat, Sapphire, had a beautiful gray coat and striking blue eyes. Sapphire would take every cracked-door advantage to escape our apartment and roam the neighborhood. It never worried me because Sapphire always made her way back home. One morning, we found Sapphire dead and I couldn't bring myself to go to school. Distraught and hysterical, my mom made a deal with me that if we found a nice burial place and had a funeral for Sapphire, I would go to school. I think showing up with a note saying I had to have a burial service for my cat before coming to school prompted my eighth grade teacher's encouragement to apply to a magnet school designed specifically for people like me: people whose love for animals was deeply embedded in our hearts.

WB Saul High School of Agricultural Sciences was a dream. It was there that I could be around what I loved the most in life: animals. I couldn't believe that there was a high school in the city of Philadelphia that had an entire farm filled with animals that I surely wouldn't find in my West Philly neighborhood. I'm talking cows, horses, pigs, sheep, beehives, small laboratory animals, and even fish.

I applied to Saul through a special admissions process, attended a summer program for incoming freshman, and happily began an experience that changed my life. Although plant and animal science were a part of the experience at Saul, I was there for one purpose only, and that was to spend as much time as possible learning all things animals.

If a cow was having difficulty delivering her calf, it was our arms going in to help her out. If the little piglets needed their razor-like teeth cut to prevent damage to their momma's nipples, we took care of that too. Saul was an experience of a lifetime. But what I thought would be the beginning of a promising future to become a veterinarian changed drastically when I became a teenage mom.

My life was twisted into an unrecognizable configuration. A positive and somewhat intact childhood, budding violinist, honors student, future veterinarian, Who's Who honoree, and the least likely to get pregnant turned into teenage motherhood. I was traumatized, to say the least, and lost—but not hopeless.

Despite my life's bleak forecast according to some, it was watching my mom demonstrate the power in rising when life knocks you down that kept me moving forward. My mom not only fortified me with a healthy foundation, but she demonstrated the power of the human spirit to rise in the face of life's adversities. I learned so much from watching my mom recover from destruction. Most importantly, I learned to never give up. This five absences rule was the first one I was planning to rise above. My mom did her best to see that her daughters made different decisions. She wanted so much for me to not experience what I was going through. The last thing she wanted was for us to become teenage mothers. Our choices were not for a lack of knowledge, because my mother taught us things about the human body, specifically female anatomy, which made us hyper-knowledgeable about ways to avoid pregnancy, the first being abstinence. When my sister and I had to sit and listen to lecture 1,001, we were busy praying the drawn-out speeches about the ovulation method, struggles of teenage pregnancy, and "boys ain't nothing but trouble" rhetoric would just end. Her threats of "this is what will happen to you if you get pregnant" alone should have scared us, but it did not.

My way of escaping pain just caused more pain. My mom wanted more than anything for her yellow and brown biscuits, her nicknames for Samira and me—to break the cycle of teenage pregnancy. She lost the battle. The one thing she fought hard to prevent, for good reasons, was the very thing that happened. My mother had a good reason for wanting a different life for her girls. She had frontline experience of what becoming a mother so early entailed. I wasn't supposed to be in the place I found myself in. I wasn't supposed to have to fight to graduate. I wasn't supposed to be facing an "F" due to five absences.

In my senior year of high school during the postpartum period after the birth of my second child, Cierra, the school counselor planned for one of my teachers to bring my homework to the house. This accommodation helped me stay on track, but it wasn't a guarantee against the rules around absences. Attending a special admissions school means you are subjected to guidelines that are not as lenient as those at regular admittance schools. My only hope was that teachers would extend a little extra grace. But there was one teacher who had a strong opinion about the course of my life. When every other teacher focused on my academic achievement and drive to succeed, he focused on the rule.

My physics teacher was going to fail me. Not because I was failing academically, but because I had missed more than five days of school. Saul had a strict rule: five absences equals a failing grade. No exceptions. Sometimes, I wonder if the rule was the real reason behind failing me. Having a baby wasn't a glamorous experience, but it felt like my physics teacher was bent on holding that against me. I was on my way to graduating, and this failing grade was going to stop that from happening. I was advised to leave the school and transfer to my neighborhood high school that would allow me to graduate despite the absences. When my daughter fell ill and I had no one to keep her, I was afraid that another absence would be the final straw on the decision to fail me.

I told my *Abi*, which means father in Arabic, what I was up against. He looked at me like he did every time I found myself in a "spilled milk" situation and said, "Let's go!"

We placed my daughter Cierra in the car seat and drove up to my school. I walked into my first period class with my books and my baby. You can imagine the silence as I sat down and placed my daughter's car seat next to my desk. I was going to graduate by any means necessary, and not from my neighborhood high school, but from the school I worked so hard to get into and stay in. I showed up. Yes, that's what I was taught to do: show up. Even when it's painful, embarrassing, and hard, show up!

My English teacher couldn't contain the shocked look on her face as I walked into class with my infant daughter in tow. With a stoic stance, I sat there knowing that if I had to walk into any class with a baby, this was the class to walk in. My English teacher was the one that came to my home after the birth of Cierra. It was one thing to visit and help me stay on track at home; it was a different situation when I showed up to class with a baby. I knew my teacher didn't have a clue as to what to do. Should she ignore the quiet baby and continue teaching? She did the next best thing and called the counselor.

My classmates were distracted, an appropriate response to bringing a baby to class. My English teacher cared about me. She didn't look at me with pity and I know she struggled over asking me to leave the class. So, she left that job for the counselor. The counselor was a sweet soul. Instead of barging into the classroom causing me to feel even more embarrassed, she just stood by the door. With the last name Abdelmalik, I was always seated at the first desk in the classroom. It was easy to find me and now it was even easier with a car seat beside me.

I explained to my counselor why I brought my daughter to school. She assured me that I would not be marked absent for the day. Staying in school, however, with my daughter was not an option. But, the counselor, my school, and the teacher who was relentless in his pursuit to fail me needed to understand that leaving to attend my neighborhood school was not an option either. I was determined to graduate in a few months. I may not have known how that was going to happen, but I knew I wasn't planning on throwing in the towel.

In ninth grade, I was smart and *cocky*. I thought my intelligence would buffer the punishment from my big mouth. I was excited about going to the "farm" school. I was in my element and excelling. For some strange reason, I thought if I was smart, it was okay to be talkative and ignore my teacher's relentless requests to be quiet. My biology teacher, however, wasn't having it. After telling me one too many times to stop talking in her class and dealing with my disrespectful responses, she set out to teach me a lesson that stuck with me for the rest of my life.

During a parent-teacher conference, my biology teacher explained to my father that she was responsible for deciding what students go on to the honors science track. Although I was one of the smartest students in the class, it was my attitude that was going to be my downfall. She further explained that she'd rather invest in a student with a better attitude than excellent grades. To say I was crushed was an understatement. My biology teacher exercised the power to change my educational journey. My teacher sought qualities in a student that went beyond good grades, and that was a lesson I never forgot.

I resented my biology teacher for what she did. My ninth grade mind couldn't grasp the fact I was the one responsible for this decision. I became both preoccupied with the power she had and a touch of paranoia. There were days when I would look outside the window of my Abi's home and see my biology teacher parked in front of the house. I was furious. Why in the world was my teacher trying to make life miserable? What would bring her to the point that she had to make house visits? *I got the lesson, now leave me alone*, I thought.

For some strange reason, although I knew it was her, my teacher never knocked on my door. One day, during a walk down my block, I saw a woman sitting on the porch at the house next door to my Abi's home. I had never seen her before. While she puffed on a cigarette, I introduced myself.

"Hi, my name is Atiya, and my dad lives next door. Did you just move here?" I asked.

She introduced herself as Shelly and said yes. She had recently relocated from Virginia with her mom, sister, and brother. I learned Shelly wasn't a grown woman. She was sixteen and sitting on the porch acting like a grown woman. Shelly and I became best friends in an instant. I shared with her my exciting school life at Saul and told her how much I loved going to the farm school, except for one major pain in my butt: my biology teacher. I went on to share how much I couldn't stand my teacher, and how she made my life miserable.

Shelly and I talked for hours. She invited me into her home and we sat looking through the pictures in her family photo albums. As Shelly flipped through the pages, I noticed a picture of my biology teacher. My next move proved that I was not as smart as I thought I was. "That's her. The one I told you about. Yeah, the teacher I can't stand," I said.

"Oh, that's my Aunt Linda. She owns the home we're living in. I'll give her a call right now," Shelly replied. I stood there in disbelief, not wanting to accept that my soon-to-be best friend was my teacher's niece. "Aunt Linda, do you have a student by the name of Atiya?"

Mortified. Yes, that pretty much sums up how I felt. *Did I just call Shelly's aunt all those names? Why didn't I look through the photo album and just keep my mouth shut? Who does that?* Well, a fourteen-year-old that learned another valuable lesson does just that. But what started out as a disaster turned into one of the biggest blessings of my life.

My biology teacher became my ally, champion, and cheerleader. When my physics teacher refused to give me a passing grade that would allow me to graduate my senior year, it was Ms. Harris, whom I eventually called with the utmost affection and gratitude, Aunt Linda, who advocated for me like nobody's business. She stood by my side and fought like a fierce Mama bear. Ms. Harris was focused on getting my physics teacher to do the right thing. In my career of leading teams, some of the most valuable lessons I passed on were not necessarily those I learned in college or in the corporate world. The lessons that carried the most meaning were the ones I learned in high school through teachers like Ms. Harris. I learned character over everything, persistence over defeat, and building relationships with unlikely heroes because you never know when you'll have to cross that bridge again. Ms. Harris taught me that it's more important to be kind, respectful, and forgiving. She taught me that when you show up differently, people will show up with you, never leaving you to fight a battle alone.

So instead of giving up or giving in, I stayed the course. I did not know until two days before my high school graduation if I was going to graduate. That anxiety-provoking experience turned into jubilation when I discovered that my physics teacher had a heart after all. I never knew the exact exchange between the two science teachers, but what I did know is that I would never accept society's limitations on my life. What I knew for sure was that God places beautiful people on Earth to do His work, and some of them are disguised as biology teachers. Ms. Harris continued to be one of my angels throughout life and Shelly and her entire family became an extension of mine.

Our graduating class sang Tevin Campbell's song, "Tomorrow." The lyrics would define the journey of my life, a journey that became a declaration. The words of the song spoke to the person who would become better, one that would never give up on their hopes or dreams, one that will show tomorrow, just how strong you will be.

I'm Not a Nurse

I WAS MORE THAN HAPPY. JUST THE MERE THOUGHT OF what I had journeyed through to experience this moment of graduating from nursing school was more than enough reason to celebrate. There were days I would sit on the trolley, with three children in tow and nursing books thick as a Webster's Dictionary, trying to study.

My mom and Abi were elated. I'm sure there was a limit on guest tickets, but when I looked back at all the pictures from that day, I know I broke the ticket limit rule. From my parents and aunts to my siblings and children, my graduation from nursing school was witnessed by so many of my loving and supportive family members. My children stared up at me with their big, brown eyes and wide smiles. I was dressed in my white nursing uniform, donning my nurse's cap while carrying the lamp of knowledge. I was also carrying peace and a great sense of accomplishment. That same tenacious spirit I had in high school, fighting for my right to graduate, propelled me through nursing school.

Nursing school was more than a notion. I took two years of prerequisite courses right after graduating high school in 1990. I was seventeen years old, living as an adult, raising my children alone in the home I spent my teenage years in. My Abi got remarried, handed me the keys to the house, but never went too far to not provide me with continued support. After two years of coursework, I entered the actual nursing program at Community College of Philadelphia. Clinicals started in the early morning, which required me to wake up in darkness to arrive on time by seven. My Abi had to travel from the Germantown section of Philadelphia to West Philadelphia in the wee hours of the morning to help transport my three children across town to make several stops at different babysitters before dropping me off at Temple Hospital. At four a.m., I'd rather toss and turn in my bed than get up and attempt to get sleepy children out the door. But, I was on a mission that some thought was impossible. There were moments on my journey when I was encouraged to not try so hard.

"You know you can stay home with your children and the government would take care of you," they'd say. I'm sure people thought they were giving me good advice, but I wanted much more for my children and me. I lost so much already, and I didn't plan on giving up after coming this far.

My nursing professor, Ivory Coleman, used to ask me what I was going to do for my parents when I graduated. She knew the trek my dad had to make on these early mornings and the sacrifices my mom made. There wasn't enough I could do for the village that got me to this point in my life. Words of gratitude wouldn't be enough, gifts could never cover it, but the way I lived my life, making the sweetest lemonade out of the lemons I was dealt would at least demonstrate that their investment and unconditional love was fully appreciated. I believe for all of us the true gift to ourselves and to others is how we live our lives.

By this time in my life, mom had pulled herself out of darkness, reclaimed her life and helped her children get about the business of living theirs. My Abi worked several jobs, always made time for family, and made sure we were okay no matter how much weight he had to carry. My bonus "step" moms helped me along various stages of my journey and were an integral part of the village that carried me. If I showed up, I could count on my family and friends, especially my six siblings to support the journey. Samira, who at times was a second mommy, encouraged and held me up when the winds of life were blowing me to bits. I owed so much to the village and decided repayment would come in the form of never giving up, no matter what.

Unlike my fellow nursing students, I didn't have a career in nursing coursing through my veins. I often listened to their stories of how deep the nursing connections were for many of them; their mothers, grand-mothers, and aunts were also nurses. They knew early on that their destiny would follow this path. This graduation moment, although special, was not the destination I had been dreaming about my entire life. Nursing was an encouraged detour, an alternate route to get me to my ultimate dream of becoming a veterinarian. Detours, roadblocks, and "closed for construction" signs were threaded throughout my young life at every intersection. I had to decide how I was going to respond, and what road I would take.

My dream was to attend Texas A&M to study pre-veterinary medicine, but my life as a young mother didn't support the idea to go away to college. My stepmother, who was both a dentist and a registered nurse, inspired my plan B. She encouraged me to apply to nursing school. Nursing would allow me to make a sufficient living, adequately provide for my children, and give me the flexibility to pursue veterinary medicine. How brilliant was this idea? I wouldn't have to struggle or rely on government assistance. I vowed that as soon as I landed a job after nursing school, my first call would be to my caseworker to tell her I would not be standing in a line ever again, collecting someone else's money. And that's exactly what I did!

I entered nursing school with a feverish excitement, but not because I'd dreamed of becoming a nurse. I was going to leverage nursing to get to my ultimate destination. I was still pretty cocky and obnoxious, but in a positive way. I was determined to succeed and create a better life, and nursing school would help me do just that.

I remember my fellow nursing students who had t-shirts that read C=RN. No, we didn't endorse "Cs," but we also knew that what we were embarking upon was no easy task. I started my nursing education at seventeen years old. Attending a community college allowed me to raise my family while pursuing my education and reach a level of self-sufficiency. Single motherhood was hard by itself. My coursework, readings, exams, and professors were not going to make it easier because of my complicated life. I had to work extra hard, study extra hard, and pray extra hard if I planned on realizing another dream, or any dream for that matter. That's just the way my life was set up; feeling bad about it and having regrets was not going to make it any better. I've had to remind myself of that often. It was that spilled milk my Abi talked about. You can't wipe it up and put back in the carton so don't waste your precious energy on something you can't change. Do better, next time.

When asked about my long lineage of nurses in the family, I found myself responding, "I only know one nurse, and she's a dentist now." Like her, nursing was not my destination. "I'm only here so I don't have to struggle while pursuing a degree in veterinary medicine," I'd explain. "You know, animals *are* kinder, gentler, and more loving creatures." Their gratefulness is instant, and their love is unconditional, something human beings have a difficult time emulating. We're mean, ungrateful, never satisfied, and selfish. I don't want to spend my life taking care of those creatures; I'd rather stick with animals.

This became my story every time someone asked me about nursing. When I repeated those words to myself, I wondered why no one ever went off on me for insulting such an admirable and heroic calling.

Dr. Tagliareni, an incredibly humble and talented nursing professor, listened to my rant about nursing being "just" a steppingstone. She was the first person that didn't accept my *truth* as truth. She would smile and say, "Atiya, you're a nurse."

I responded, "Maybe, but only for a moment." I had big plans, and my respect and admiration for Dr. Tagliareni was not going to change *those* plans. But I've always heard it said, "If you want to make God laugh, make plans."

I wanted to become a veterinarian. That was my purpose. I was afraid of letting that dream go. It was the last part of my dream that I wanted so strongly to hold onto. I loved animals and there weren't enough detours that would take me from that destination. I was holding on, yes, for dear life and these nursing students and professors weren't going to take that away from me. The decisions I made had robbed me of enough.

The beauty of nursing school is that you get to rotate through various disciplines. This served several purposes, including providing a well-rounded approach to training and exposure to various specialty areas such as psychiatric, geriatric, pediatric, and labor and delivery nursing.

I found out early that I was good at therapeutic communication, a way of communicating to get the maximum benefit from the nurse-patient relationship. I was also afforded great opportunities to practice this form of communication during my psychiatric nursing rotation. But just because you're good at something doesn't necessarily mean you're passionate about it. I had enough of my own issues to deal with; I couldn't imagine carrying the weight of someone else's. No, I wasn't a nurse, and I definitely wasn't a psychiatric nurse.

During the labor and delivery rotation, unlike other clinical settings, student nurses wore the same scrub uniforms as "real" nurses. This was both good and bad. Good because wearing the same scrubs created the illusion that you were the real deal, bad because you could be mistaken for one.

The bad experience of wearing the same scrubs changed my life forever when I was tasked with acting like real nurse. Our nursing class was on the labor and delivery rotation at Pennsylvania Hospital, located in the historic downtown section of Philadelphia. I was assigned to a patient in active labor. The "real" nurse gave me specific instructions: "Sit close to the monitor. All you need to focus on is this top line right here. This is the baby's heartbeat. It's okay if it dips, but that dip needs to bounce back up. If the dip stays down, be concerned, and call for me immediately," she said.

My mouth and head nodded in agreement, but in my mind, I was giving her the side-eye look. The conversation in my head went something like this: *Are you serious? You're going to leave me in this room, with this woman who is in extreme discomfort, and without any support except for me, a scared-to-death nursing student?*

None of those thoughts came out of my mouth, but inside I felt it needed to be said. I was scared.

There was another life besides the one in front of me, one that had not made it to the world, one for whom I was also responsible. I needed to be fully present. I was reminded in this moment of Ms. Harris' lesson to keep my mouth shut. This was one of those moments.

I sat there in front the "freaking" machine that was accurately known as an external fetal monitor. I did one of my dog Nemo's numbers that I call *acting invisible*. This happens when he stands extremely still and looks at you through the corner of his guilt-ridden eyes as if to say, "I'm not really here. You really don't see me, and I'm not responsible for the ripped-up trash bag."

I stared at the monitor while trying my best to be there for a patient going through an experience I was all too familiar with: Bringing life into the world. I was a mom myself by then, three times, but it's a totally different experience when you watch someone else go through the stages of childbirth.

The obstetrician showed up and asked about his patient's progress. He barked orders to get him a pair gloves so he could check to see how far she was dilated. I was a nervous wreck. I wanted out of that room so bad! The invisible Nemo trick didn't work, and neither did pretending I was on an episode of *Star Trek*, where beaming to another place was an option.

"She's ready. Baby's crowning." The obstetrician gave me that update with the expectation that I was going to do something with that information. This was my first day in labor and delivery, and, as nervous as I was, hopefully my last.

The stress I felt was overwhelming. Besides, I had plans to become a veterinarian anyway. Having that level of responsibility for a new life was heavy, heroic, and life-changing.

The "real" nurse's entrance into the room was perfect timing. I was enveloped by a sense of calm, and the mommy instinct kicked in. The baby's head was crowning and instead of shying away from the experience, I jumped in full-force and stood at "my" patient's bedside, holding her hand and coaching her to breathe and push. I witnessed a human

being bring another human being into the world, and at that moment
Dr. Tagliareni was proven right. I was a nurse.

Denied

AS A NURSE, I WAS CONFRONTED BY THE FRACTURED WORLD of health care every single time I stepped foot into the small community hospital where I spent much of my clinical career. My patients often showed up in the frailest forms, both young and old. I witnessed first-hand the ill effects of living in an environment where socioeconomic status weighed heavily on all aspects of health.

Like in many urban dwellings, access to a safe area to play and engage in physical activity, and food that fueled a healthy body were scarce commodities in my neighborhood. Instead, stores were stocked with boxes of processed foods and shelves of penny candy secured behind Plexiglass, just low enough for kids to see, causing them to pull on their mother's coattails while they begged, whined, and performed tricks to get enough junk to rot their stomachs away. Undesirable corner stores and playgrounds with broken equipment and tattered basketball hoops could be found in urban neighborhoods across our city. Many of our communities were not built to build families up. Life became an exercise in survival, and while we appeared to survive, I can't say we were doing a good job of thriving.

It was no surprise to see my patients in the worst state of health. I started as a night shift nurse on a hematology/oncology floor and took care of cancer patients, patients with blood disorders, and a myriad of other conditions. This hospital, like other hospitals, was a place where many people came to die rather than to be healed.

This was especially true when caring for patients with cancer. As a night shift nurse, I rarely witnessed those patients do well and survive to

A LIFE WORTH SAVING

tell the tale of beating cancer. Many of them were at the end of life and knew it. I'll never forget the night an older gentleman was admitted with an advanced stage of cancer. During the admission process, I worked feverishly to get him as comfortable as possible. I tried to convince him to change into a hospital gown, but he refused. He just wanted to lie in bed in his own clothes.

After getting him settled, I started his IV medications and left the room to gather additional items. While sitting at the nurse's station, the nursing assistant approached me and said she didn't think my patient was breathing. As I ran back into the room, I knew what I would face: my patient, breathless. The beeping sound from the machines was the only noise invading the cold, lifeless room. I immediately called a CODE and began the resuscitation process. With the first chest compression came a geyser-like eruption of the diseased, green contents from his stomach.

This became a normal, frequent existence for me. I didn't enjoy becoming so familiar with death. More than a decade later, I still remember him and so many others whose lives were wrecked by disease. Many that could have been prevented if managed effectively, treated early, and given an opportunity for full healing.

I worked the night shift for two years before experiencing a burnout of the heart. I remember my fellow nurses telling me that I would get used to it. The weight of the pain in watching so many in *pain* would slide off my shoulders and going from one resuscitation to the next wouldn't affect me as much. I waited patiently for the moment to be free of the pain, but soon came to the realization that I wasn't designed that way.

I was wired to feel. I didn't understand it back then, but now I know that who I am is a part of my purpose, and to fully live *in* my purpose, I must *feel*. I spent a lot of time caring for others in both my professional and personal life. It hit me hard when I found out that my life was in just as much need of caring and healing.

I guess I had to thank the life insurance company for denying my application. Without that denial, I may have walked around for a long time before my kidneys were damaged enough, since it's possible to lose up to ninety percent of your kidney function before exhibiting symptoms. Early detection was one of my biggest blessings.

Applying for a life insurance policy was my attempt as a single mother to financially protect my three children. What I didn't realize at the time was that the best life insurance policy against disability and premature death were the daily choices that would facilitate health and healing. I'd fought to escape the healthy lifestyle that represented the foundation of my childhood, and in that moment, it hit me so hard what my mom tried to do. She wasn't punishing her children; she was trying to save us.

All this time, I thought I was healthy, even years after abandoning my "Earth Family" lifestyle. But one word—*denied*—changed that healthy illusion in the blink of an eye. Additional lab tests and a kidney biopsy revealed focal segmental glomerulosclerosis, a filtration disease of the kidneys. This condition prevented my kidneys from working as the washing machine of the body. I was informed that within five years, I would most likely be on dialysis and a transplant list. I was offered two medication options: steroids or methotrexate, a drug used in the treatment of cancer and other diseases. I'm a nurse, and like many of us, we know too much.

I decided to take my own option, called "wait and see," and continue to visit the nephrologist and get my scheduled lab work as ordered. I learned a year later that "wait and see" was not a good option either. That option was going to lead to my destiny with dialysis and the transplant list much sooner than five years.

The lab tests were revealing progression in my disease state. After much thought and research, I decided to take the treatment option that I thought was the lesser of the two evils. It didn't take long for me to realize that the fine print of side effects found on prescriptions are real.

Worrying will kill us prematurely, stop us from living, and have us always assuming the worst. In her book, *Making it Happen*, Lara Casey shares the irony in worrying. She refers to it as if we're praying for something we don't want to happen—and I was becoming a pro at it.

As a single mom, I worried about everything. Not only did I worry, but my mind would invent the most horrific scenarios. If my kids were late getting home, my first thought was, *who kidnapped my babies?* I wasn't thinking they were simply taking their time to walk home from school, or that my youngest was doing the usual by giving his older siblings a hard time. No, it had to be a psychopath camped outside of the school waiting for the perfect opportunity to grab all three of my children, stuff them in a car, and hold them for ransom. That was an irrational thought for more than one reason. Mainly, a would-be kidnapper would have picked the wrong neighborhood to take a child and expect that someone would have money to pay a ransom.

In my normal worrier fashion, the first thing I did after receiving the infamous insurance denial letter was assume the absolute worst. I began planning my funeral and praying my three children wouldn't have to be separated after my death. My mom was not one of those grandmothers who would jump at the opportunity to babysit, so asking her to raise three kids was a stretch.

It wasn't a question of love, because she surely loved her grandchildren, but my mom got her grandchildren fix in ten minutes or less. For the first five minutes, she's hugging and kissing, and the next five she's thanking us for stopping by and ushering us out the door. She was on the list of people to raise my children in my absence, but she wasn't at the top of that list.

After planning my funeral, I decided that I wasn't ready to give up, and that I needed to call my friend, an oncologist/hematologist I worked with at the hospital. My calls to him were usually about his patients and the miserable fact that they died on my shift. He would often remind he was a cancer doctor and to pull myself together. Not all outcomes would be good.

Well, I never got used to that explanation, and I did not grow thick skin as he and my fellow nurses said would happen. I explained the results of the extensive testing I had done for the insurance policy and the subsequent denial letter. After talking me off the ledge, he referred me to a nephrologist. And so, began my new life with kidney disease.

Why Me?

I COULDN'T SEE THE CLOCK! AT ONE OF THE MOST CRITICAL moments in my job, the clock was a blurry vision that might as well have been non-existent. I panicked as I quickly moved close enough to see the numbers while I transported the newborn to the warming bed.

Within my job, unlike what occurred in my life, I wanted precision and perfection. I did not want to fail at not being exact on the time of birth. It may sound superficial, but I knew as a mom and labor and delivery nurse that the time of birth was something that would be shared for this baby's entire lifetime.

The blurry vision was a sign, but it wasn't the only one I had ignored. The fact that I drank gallons of water followed by two-liter bottles of orange soda in a day without even coming close to quenching my thirst was yet another sign. The vanity in me was the most likely culprit responsible for the delay in alerting my kidney doctor to the symptoms I was experiencing. I lost a lot of weight in a short period, so my journey to skinny was now being realized. It's unbelievable at times to think of how far I was willing to go to reach what I thought would make me happy in life. To me, it was being skinny again! It's also amazing how far we'll go to save someone else's life before we go to great lengths to save our own. My life didn't become worthy to save until the symptoms threatened my ability to perform my job of helping others.

The insurance denial letter set off a chain reaction that led me to battling a disease they didn't give me much hope in beating. I had been on prednisone for kidney disease for one month when the symptoms started to appear. The thirst and the drastic weight loss were telltale signs that I was having a severe reaction to the medication. I was hesitant to try either of the two treatments presented to me after being diagnosed. As a nurse, I've administered both treatment options to patients and was well-versed on their side effects. Remember, it took a year before I consented to choosing what I thought was the lesser of the two evils. Now, with blurred vision and unquenchable thirst, I questioned my decision and tried desperately not to worry if my life was at stake.

Attending to the newborn included noting the correct time of birth, performing the APGAR assessment (a critical test that scores how well the baby is adjusting to life outside the womb), and administering newborn medications. I wrapped the newborn in a warm and cozy blanket and placed her in her happy but exhausted mother's arms. I rushed out of the room with a sense of urgency that it was now time for me to treat my own life like a precious gift. After explaining my symptoms, my doctor ordered stat labs, which are supposed to mean "right now." Life has taught me that words don't necessarily translate into action. Although it took a minute to draw my stat labs, the processing took what felt like an eternity. Instead of waiting around for the results, I made the not-so-smart decision to drive the hour-long commute to my new suburban home in Downingtown, Pennsylvania.

Deep down inside, I knew I wasn't in any condition to drive. What made me come up with this genius plan, especially after being overly upset and panicky because I couldn't see the clock? For some strange reason, I felt I was suddenly healed and okay enough to drive on the road, at night, with other cars. I know what you're thinking. *Real smart.*

Prior to moving to Downingtown, I lived and worked in the same neighborhood where I had lived since I was fifteen years old. A two-minute commute to work turned into an hour on a good day. Working non-traditional shifts, like seven a.m. to seven p.m., helped avoid the dreaded traffic that often made me feel like my primary residence was a box with windows on four wheels. On those days it felt like my car was planted in one spot more than in motion like it was designed for.

Apart from my vision loss and desert-like thirst, I had a pretty good night helping women bring their babies into the world. I said to myself, *if something were terribly wrong with my labs, someone would surely call me.* But did I really need a call to tell me to stay put? The decision to get behind the wheel of my car was proof that I was ignoring all the calls my body was trying to make to my disconnected brain. In pure Atiya fashion, I decided to go to the mall, shop, and have dinner—while drinking another two gallons of liquids—instead of driving straight home. It was a great idea at the time since I wanted some "me" time before I walked into the house with my children clamoring for my attention. Since I successfully made it to the mall and dinner without causing any accidents, I thought I wasn't as sick as I felt. But with the continued thirst and eyes that were playing tricks on me, I knew deep down all was not well. Still, despite the facts and the darkness that consumed the road, I got back in the car.

I saw the two tractor-trailers headed directly toward me. The size of the trucks alone had caught my attention. The only problem, and perhaps the biggest one, was that I couldn't tell which lanes the trucks were in. *Was I on the wrong side of the road? Was it really two trucks, or was my vision so blurry that I couldn't clearly make out what was in front of me?*

I had to make a split-second decision as the trucks quickly approached. A decision that ultimately saved my life. I quickly swerved my car to the right, hopped the curb, and landed with the front of my car halfway on the side of the road. On top of not being able to see clearly, my heart felt like it was beating outside of my chest. I was close to the subdivision I lived in, so I reassembled my panic-stricken body, slowly backed off the side of the road, and made it home.

No, I didn't call for help or alarm Mike, my boyfriend I shared a home with. Pride and embarrassment were not positive additions to my already fear-filled, injured ego. I knew that the decision to drive home was an irresponsible one, and the added stop to shop and eat made me feel even worse. I made it safely to my driveway, but as soon as I got to the top of the steps, I was greeted with the news from Mike that sent my life into a tailspin.

She's Alive

I FELT MORE LIKE A SPECTACLE THAN A PATIENT. IN A teaching hospital, you get to be the subject of study for everyone, including residents, medical students, and a whole slew of others. The only thing you can do while lying half-naked with what feels like a thin layer of cheap material tied in two places, is try to remain calm and polite as you answer the same questions over and over.

Being a patient allowed me to see how it felt on the other side. Like many healthcare professionals, if you have enough sense and compassion when the tables get turned, the experience will help you be a more compassionate clinician—or better yet, human being. The medical residents found it quite amazing that I was still alert despite my dire stat lab results. They poked their heads into my curtained space in the emergency room as if to say, "Wow, she's alive."

My blood sugar was over 1100, an unfortunate and tragic response to the medical treatment that was designed to save, not harm me. I guess I was the victim of the words that are spoken so fast at the end of a drug commercial. You know the ones that tell you you're at risk of dying while they display a picture of someone having the time of their lives, holding hands with the love of their lives, and strolling across the beach. Well, the drug treatment I chose backfired and brought the meaning of the fine print to life.

The medical term was just as scary to pronounce: steroid-induced hyperglycemic hyperosmolar nonketotic coma, or, to keep it simple, HHNK, a metabolic emergency that could induce a coma, or worse, when left untreated. I learned about my condition while lying in a cold room under bright lights, which illuminated my irresponsible decision to not wait for my stat lab results. My kidney doctor had called my home to deliver the message that the results indicated I was facing a life-threatening condition. As he ended his instructions on which hospital to bring me to, his final words to Mike were, "I just pray she's not behind the wheel of a car."

I begged the nurse to allow me to use the restroom instead of having a Foley catheter placed, because it was a reminder that I was losing control over my life and being admitted to the Intensive Care Unit (ICU) didn't provide an ounce of comfort. The nurse looked at me as if she was thinking, *You're a nurse. What part of this conversation don't you understand?*

Lord knows the last thing I wanted was a rubber tube coming out of me, draining urine into a bag that would eventually be hung on the side of my bed, like a purse on one of those hangers you find neatly tucked under a restaurant table. If my night didn't contain enough excitement, I would now have to resign myself to the fact that I was indeed sick. And not just a little sick, but admitted-to-the-ICU kind of sick. My symptoms—including the high blood sugar, blurry vision, unquenchable thirst, and drastic and quick weight loss—were bright, flashing warning signs that I needed to proceed with caution and quickly find a detour to save my life. Maybe I did understand how sick I was, but I was too afraid to face the reality of what was happening. *Why Me?*

Triumph

THEY STARED LONG AND HARD AS I ENTERED THE GROUP session of the program. I'm sure the look on my face conveyed both curiosity and uncertainty. I didn't feel like I belonged during that first encounter, but I felt like no matter what was in store, this part of my journey was exactly where I needed to be. The *Dr. Dean Ornish Program for Reversing Heart Disease* was my "end of the rope" chance to save my life.

In January 2005, I began my career at Highmark Blue Cross Blue Shield, a major health plan headquartered in Pittsburgh, Pennsylvania. Six months prior, I had relocated from Philadelphia with my children in tow to live happily ever after with my friend turned fiancé, a physician who I met at a hospital where I worked in Philadelphia. His new position at one of the community hospitals in western Pennsylvania required us to move five hours from the comfort of the familiar and the people I loved dearly. I didn't relocate under the best conditions. The original plan was for me to take the LSAT and pursue a career in healthcare law. Those plans abruptly changed when my fiancé asked me to move to Pittsburgh sooner rather than later. Waiting for me to finish school and trying to navigate the distance between us would be a bit much for a young marriage, so I agreed. We were friends that became on and off partners. We had worked in the same community hospital, where I spent most of my clinical career. We read scripture together, traveled and shopped together, and did what besties do. I moved reluctantly, and my children even more reluctantly.

Happily ever after became one of the most challenging and disheartening experiences of my life. Our bestie relationship transitioned into two people fighting to keep love alive, but failing miserably at it. We were great friends and should have cherished what we did best: friendship. Instead, we tried to merge two distinct personalities and ways of being into one cohesive family unit. The differences were irreconcilable.

The decision to call off my wedding after having two showers, relocating, and leaving what I knew best—my family and friends—was both brave and bold. *What would I do now?* I thought. *How would I sustain our lives without a job and no support system?* I worried about what the world would think of my decision. I started out by calling my mother for a much-needed pep talk and guidance. My primary concern was deciding whether or not to go through with the wedding even though I knew it wasn't the right decision for all parties. My mom, who I considered my very own oracle, spent no time ushering my mind from pity and defeat to planning and victory. She told me that my decision wasn't about anyone else. This was *my* life I was talking about, and for that reason alone I needed to make a choice that was best for my children and me.

The stress of my crumbling personal life and present chronic conditions was surely a recipe for disaster. I came to what I thought was the only logical conclusion, and that was to move back home where I would be surrounded by love, support, a career, and all things familiar. I contacted Americhoice of Pennsylvania, my former employer in Philadelphia and was not only offered my job back, but given the choice of two positions to consider. I contacted a moving company and informed my family and friends that I was on my way back home. The feeling of hopelessness and confusion was lifted as everything seemed to fall into place. I only had to endure this unknown place, Pittsburgh, for thirty more days. Nothing made me more excited than the thought of being home where an abundance of unconditional love awaited.

But that phrase popped up again: *if you ever want to make God laugh, make plans.*

As everything seemed to fall into place, I decided that what I needed more than ever was to continue to go to church during my final thirty days in Pittsburgh. The easy route would have been to stay put in the house until my departure to Philadelphia. But I knew that wallowing in pity and embarrassment would only make things worse. Continued check-ins with my loved ones gave me enough positive energy to get up and keep it moving until the time came to head down the PA Turnpike into safe territory. In the time I had left, I needed to find a source of comfort. I yearned for a spiritual revival of the soul. I remembered hearing a pastor from Pittsburgh preach at my home church in Philadelphia, Enon Tabernacle. At the end of his sermon, he invited anyone to come visit Mt. Ararat Baptist Church, if we were ever in Pittsburgh. I wasn't very familiar with the city since my ex-fiancé wasn't fond of me traveling outside of our comfortable suburban environment. Making the trek to Mt. Ararat reminded me of my rebellious and determined nature and it gave my spirit the boost it needed, even if it was temporary. I wasn't a stranger to hard stuff; I was just getting tired of it.

The morning of my first visit was eventful. It started with a straight trek down Route 65 with my youngest son in tow. All was well until we found ourselves a tad bit lost near the church. I was close, but not close enough. I saw a big red sign that read, "Buses Only," but for some strange reason, I turned on the route anyway. Wrong decision. The familiar sound of a police cruiser's siren was a strong indication that the route was truly for buses only, and that my little red car missed that description by a long shot. Fear filled my spirit as I pulled to the side of the road. This feeling was a far cry from the peace and sanctuary I was seeking in the comfort of church.

The officer must have seen the panic splashed across my face because he lightened the encounter with a head tilted smile and asked, "You aren't from around here, are you?"

"Officer, you're right," I replied. "I'm lost and trying to find my way to Mt. Ararat Baptist Church." A wave of relief rushed through me as the officer let me go with a warning *and* directions to get to the church. Before I pulled off, I also hoped he could give me more than just directions. I wanted so desperately to ask if he had any advice on getting the rest of my life on the right road. I decided to keep that inquiry to myself. I didn't want to give the officer any reason to give me more than a warning. The headlines wouldn't read well: "Single mom drives on 'Buses Only' route with frightened son in tow; asks police officer for directions on how to get her life back on track."

After arriving at Mt. Ararat, my son and I enjoyed a great service and wonderful fellowship. On the way home, my son respectfully asked if we could find a church closer to home, one that would not require us driving through bus-only routes. Since I hadn't planned on staying in Pittsburgh for more than a month, I had no problem spending each Sunday at a different church. The next weekend, while my son was in Philadelphia spending time with family, I decided to attend St. Matthews church in Sewickley, Pennsylvania. It was a quick and safe five-minute drive from my home with no bus-only routes. Immediately following service, I was invited to join the women at a luncheon in the lower sanctuary of the church. I engaged in a conversation with a pleasant older woman, and I now strongly believe she was placed in my life as a guide to getting me on the life-saving road I'd been seeking.

Like most new encounters I experienced in Pittsburgh, I was asked the same question: "What's your story?" Everyone I met wanted to know why I was here, where I came from, and where was I headed.

As I shared what I could bear sharing without bursting into tears, the woman encouraged me to visit Triumph Baptist Church in Sewickley, just a few blocks from St. Matthews. The older woman didn't say much, but the message was in her eyes. She said that Triumph would be a great place for me and my family. She didn't explain why, after only one encounter with me, she knew where I belonged. But it was the unspoken exchange between us that gave me the most comfort and assurance that I should just listen and heed her advice. Triumph would be the third stop on my church tour.

At the time, Triumph Baptist Church was situated right outside of Pittsburgh in the town of Sewickley. The church greets you at the corner of a residential block filled with giant trees and country porches.

Triumph reminded me of the small family churches back home in Philadelphia. It was a welcoming, but not overwhelming, sight. It appears Triumph intentionally avoided the megachurch syndrome, making it an unintimidating place for a lost soul like me.

I knew I brought my own weight of anxiety, and I was not looking forward to being met with stares from strangers trying to figure out who I was and why I came to their church. But with its historic character intact, stained-glass windows and old-fashioned pews, I immediately felt like I was in a room full of extended family members; you know the kind you meet at family reunions and spend the day tracing your family tree to connect the branches? I felt the energy as soon as I walked into the vestibule.

The melodic sounds of instruments and the choir singing greeted me as I entered the double doors that led to the sanctuary. A large crowd filled every single pew of the small, humble church. I later learned that the crowded and festive energy in the room was attributed to a special occasion: the pastor's twentieth anniversary. I was met with smiles from everyone I walked by as I made my way to a seat in the back pew. I immediately felt a sense of comfort and relief. For the first time in weeks, I felt myself breathe. Although my spirit was unsettled, this moment allowed me to be enveloped by a haven, a place that I needed so much in my life. Amid "hallelujahs," "amens," clapping, and stomping feet, I felt like my mind was sifting through the events of the past few months. I tried hard to come to grips with what I was experiencing, but everything seemed so surreal.

Why wasn't I with my fiancé preparing for our upcoming nuptials? I thought. *Where were my children? And why am I sitting in this church, with people I had absolutely no connection with?* I felt like I had a terrible case of whiplash as I sat there trying to thread the pieces of my life back together. I felt like I would gain some sense of comfort if I could put one piece of the puzzle together again. Relocating back to a place of safety, familiarity and family is what I thought I needed to begin the healing process. I looked forward to being surrounded by family and friends that wouldn't try to figure out my story by staring, or even worse, to claim they knew it by my false appearance. I'd mastered the art of illusion. Yes, I looked like everything was intact, but one of the biggest misconceptions is reading a book by its cover. Going home wasn't going to answer all the lingering questions as to how I'd gotten myself into this in the first place, but at least home would be a place where my journey wouldn't be a lonely one.

Toward the end of the sermon, the pastor opened the doors of the church for anyone who wanted to join. I felt someone lift me up out of the pew and push me toward the aisle. The only problem with what I thought happened and what actually happened was that no one was there to push me. At this point, with the recent tornado-like events of my life, I was beginning to feel like I needed an intervention. Because nothing else could explain why I suddenly stood up in a church full of strangers and walk down the aisle to join a church, in a city I was about to leave.

Dr. Taglarieni, my psychiatric nursing professor, was right when she said, "All behavior is meaningful and purposeful no matter how it may appear to you." I guess I was fully realizing the truth in those words because I was either seriously losing my mind or my journey to save my life was being answered. If that was the case, this was a strange answer. Without turning my head to look at each side of the church, I knew without a shadow of a doubt that everyone was staring at me. I silently asked myself, *are you losing it?* And, I was dead serious.

Why else would I walk down the aisle to join a church when I had no intentions of making this place home? Thank goodness, those thoughts only raced through my mind behind a plastic smile. My next thought was, *if you're really listening, I need help and I'm hoping walking down this aisle will get me there or at least closer!* It truly felt like an out-of-body experience. I felt I had no control over my actions. My mind quickly flashed back to the conversation I had with the older woman at St. Matthews one week ago: *Triumph is where you need to be.* This was getting a little spooky. Step by step, as I walked up the aisle, I felt stares and soft whispers. There were days like this that I felt my story was written all over my face.

In that moment, I knew there was no turning back. I knew that all the great plans to return home were drastically changed with this one decision. I knew that this walk down the aisle was not simply to join a church; it was the Holy Spirit ushering me. With a called-off wedding, three hundred miles from family and friends, my children and I would embark on an adventure, an unplanned journey to a destination yet to be discovered.

These Four Things

WHEN MOST FOLKS WOULD ATTEST TO THEIR JOBS BEING A source of misery and death, mine played a significant role in saving my life. It was because of my job that I landed in the Ornish program, four months after making the decision to make a life in Pittsburgh. Highmark is a progressive health and wellness company that pioneered wellness initiatives long before they were considered sexy. The leadership role the company took when it came to cultivating and providing the resources to live a healthy life was a primary reason why I chose to work at the company despite being offered a higher salaried job at another health care organization. I knew I needed more than a paycheck. I needed a living that would support the journey to save my life. On the day of my interview, I walked past the company's fitness center. Seeing the bright, airy, and welcoming facility put an extra pep in my step and a smile on my face. During the interview, I made sure to ask the typical questions, but I also included questions about how the company invested in the health and well-being of its employees.

For once in my life, I could make a living, and money would not be my primary reason for accepting a job. I knew that money couldn't save my life. I understood that the chronic conditions I lived with didn't care about my title or salary. If the conditions had their way, I wouldn't be able to make a living for long because their goal was to tear me apart, limb by limb. I felt good about my decision to accept the job offer at Highmark. I didn't know all the resources that would become available from this opportunity, but having a gym in the same building I worked in was one more item I was able to check off the master plan to get my life right.

One of the programs offered by Highmark included the *Know Your Numbers* campaign. This initiative focused on biometric screenings that provided you with tangible information, including your blood glucose (sugar), blood pressure, weight/Body Mass Index, and cholesterol. In addition to knowing your numbers, participants filled out a health assessment that provided an evaluation that went underneath the plastic smile, great wardrobe, and snazzy shoes. Being a willing participant in the screening and health assessment was the trigger for a special invitation to be evaluated for participation in the Dr. Dean Ornish's Program for Reversing Heart Disease.

While going through the mail on one sunny afternoon, I came across an envelope from Highmark. The letter read like one of those sweepstakes announcements that make you believe you've won one million dollars and a host of other prizes. It reminded me of the days when the Ed McMahon commercials would show him knocking on some lucky, surprised hometown American's door to present them with an oversized check intended to change their lives.

My letter was earth-shattering in a different way. I never imagined myself saying this, but reading that letter felt better than an announcement that I had won the sweepstakes. That letter was far more important than money because it contained information that could literally save my life. Money, regardless of how much I love to shop, was no match for my life. I wanted to live like nobody's business. Not just get by, but thrive amid conditions that were doing their best to take me down. I held the secret, in my hands, to become my own superhero. No drugs. No gimmicks. No joke.

As I read the letter line by line, a sense of hope and curiosity flooded my thoughts. My mind began to wander, and it led me on this imaginary "Little Atiya" journey of what life would be like if I weren't consumed by the constant threat of death from my illnesses. Three words from the title alone, *Reversing Heart Disease*, were enough for me to imagine the possibility of not being afraid of diabetes, kidney disease, and all its ugliness. *Was this even possible? Was this a joke?* I thought. There were no pills, clinical trials, or magic potions mentioned in the letter, so how in the world could my lifestyle alone have that much power to reverse disease? At that point in my life, I didn't have the luxury of not taking advantage of every opportunity to save myself. I wasn't going to be the one sitting back and wishing I had taken that first step.

The letter contained an invitation to participate in a life-changing program offered at select hospitals across the city. I decided to call the Allegheny General Hospital location. This location was close to the office and the closest to my home. I was at least going to pick up the phone and interrogate the poor soul on the other end with relentless questions as to how the heck living this lifestyle could save my life. Dr. Ornish spent many years proving this truth, proving his naysayers, fellow colleagues, and others wrong. People do have that kind of power. Everything needed to change the trajectory of our lives is in our hands. They say people will make time for what's important. You can come up with a million excuses. But if you really—and I mean *really*—want something, you'll make it happen.

I had nothing to lose. Yes, the Ornish program was a huge commitment that required me to spend four hours twice a week going through all four components of the program. After explaining to my three children, who were in high school and middle school at the time, the program's possibility to change my health, there was no doubt I had the support to go for it. The Dr. Dean Ornish Program for Reversing Heart Disease is made up of four components, all needed to save your life: a whole foods nutrition plan, stress management, group support, and exercise. The program components combined were proven to reverse heart disease and a whole host of other chronic conditions. So, although I wasn't diagnosed with heart disease, the diseases I was battling were co-conspirators and could be taken down by participating in the program.

Group support, a moment for social connectedness, was a time for the participants to convene in a period of reflection, support, and healing. You were kindly asked to check judgment and advice at the door. Lord knows if we had all the answers, the sessions would be empty. Upon walking into my first group session, it was clear that I was the youngest Ornish participant. Like most people who are shocked once I share my laundry list of chronic conditions, they, too, looked at me like I was sent as a spy and not simply one of them.

For most older people I've encountered, filtering words was clearly a thing of the past. This group of older participants was no different. Eventually, the group's silent consensus to remain nonjudgmental was broken. "What could possibly be wrong with you?" asked an older, gentle-looking woman. I guess between the silent stares, she became the chosen one to speak up and ask me—the imposter—why I was there. "You don't look like you belong," the woman continued. There are millions of people walking around with illnesses that you can't see. Would I be treated differently if I walked around with a sign that said: "Diabetes, high blood pressure, high cholesterol, low vitamin D, chronic knee pain, chronic back pain, migraines, and kidney disease"?

Would someone make a different choice because they could read what was happening in my life? Would someone walk up to me and say, "You know you should probably choose the apple instead of the donut." Or, "Maybe you should walk up these stairs instead of waiting for the elevator." Telling me that I looked like I didn't belong further reinforced the misconception that people believe you must have a certain look when you're sick. Two words: Halle Berry. She's one person who clearly doesn't look like she's battling diabetes. And I'm proof that there isn't a certain look, and that I probably had more reasons to be sitting there than many others, even the older group members. My pillbox looked like a mini suitcase. No, I didn't look sick on the outside, but I had already mastered the art of disguise. Looking good not only hid the evidence of my chronic illnesses, but it also covered up the broken spirit that continually searched for healing.

The healing never lasted because it wasn't built upon true spiritual transformation and self-love. It was the rush of shopping to at least look like I was all right. It was the plastic smile that hid the pain. It was the overachiever that made sure everything else in her life was all right, even when the most important pieces were falling apart. Yes, I belonged right here in this group with the rest of them trying to hold onto a piece of hope, an opportunity to reverse the diseases that invaded my body.

On program night, the group journeyed through each hour-long module of stress management, group support, exercise, and a whole foods dinner together. Each lived experience in the program allowed us to learn how to live this lifestyle on our own. We were being shown a way of living that produced life. The proof was in the biometric results taken after twelve weeks in the program that clearly showed a dramatic decrease in all my numbers, including weight, blood pressure, and blood sugar. The Ornish program has proven that these four components combined can reverse heart disease. And because there's clear evidence that heart disease is not the only condition that's impacted by lifestyle, the program has proven to reduce or eliminate other illnesses and literally change the trajectory of your life.

Dr. Ornish also developed the Spectrum program for those who think the Ornish program is too hard or don't want to live that lifestyle. The Spectrum offers just that: a spectrum of options that will give you flexibility, but still help you make choices on your journey to live your best life. Going through the Ornish program felt like my own version of the prodigal son story. Each component closely resembled the foundation my mother laid for us in our early childhood. As a young girl, we practiced yoga and meditated. Lack of exercise was not a problem for our Earth Family, and the nutrition plan was right up my mom's alley. A vegetarian lifestyle was our way of living. Social connectedness was our way of thriving. Before Ornish proved that doing these four things could reverse heart disease, my mother conducted her own study. Not because she had something to prove, but because she loved her children so much she wanted them to live, and live abundantly.

I remember the day I told my mom about the Ornish program. In pure Karima fashion, she asked if I was kidding: "Oh, now you're going to listen to that doctor instead of what your momma was telling you all along?" I told my mom to think of the Ornish program as a "welcome home." My life drastically changed following the program. Every condition I battled was being defeated.

The biggest problem with anything that requires behavior change is sustainability. What happens when life happens? How do you respond when the joy ride turns into being thrown off the train? It became harder and harder to be consistent. I wasn't just on a yo-yo diet; I was on a yo-yo life. But I kept getting back up. I fed myself the same messages I found so easy to feed others, including my patients, family, friends, and complete strangers. I was always encouraging and speaking life into someone else's existence. I wanted to believe the words I deposited into others, and I wanted my life to reflect that I also internalized them. I believed that no matter what, you get up. That no matter how hard things are, you get up. That no matter how many times you fall, you get up, and you keep it moving as if your life depended on it. Because it does. I just needed my belief to last long enough for there to be absolutely no reason, no event, no life's happenings that could knock me off the path.

A Broken Heart Still Beats

WHEN I MOVED TO PITTSBURGH, I ENJOYED THE ADVEN-
ture of visiting various parts of the city and surrounding areas. The
topography alone intrigued me. I moved from the relatively flat city
of Philadelphia, which was filled with the excitement of a big town, to
a much smaller city that included hills, mountains, bridges, and rivers.

Upon our arrival in Pittsburgh, I remember my youngest son saying,
"Mom, there are houses built into the hills." It was startling to see such
a sight, which sparked a curiosity about the town that we would soon
call our second home.

I didn't hesitate to travel to various parts of Pittsburgh, including
Shadyside, East Liberty, North Hills, and Mt. Washington. This kind of
travel was normal for us because our family and friends were spread out
over Philadelphia, the surrounding suburbs, and South Jersey.

But I found the vibe in Pittsburgh to be much different. When I
shared the details of my city excursions with my new acquaintances, I
was often met with a puzzled expression followed by, "You went where?"

It didn't take long to figure out that the bridges, tunnels, and rivers
clearly separated Pittsburghers, and traveling just to take a ride wasn't
their cup of tea. I realized that most folks did everything on their side
of town. The unspoken motto was, "If I lived in the North, then I stayed
in the North."

One of my trips took me to Homestead, the waterfront area of the
city. Besides being the shopping area, this section of town reminded me
of an old western town with abandoned storefronts and old signs, rem-
nants of what looked like a vibrant place in its heyday. Once a bustling

steel mill town that received international attention for the violent Homestead strike, the area is now lined with historic buildings and a waterfront shopping center, which of course, is my favorite attraction.

Being new to the area didn't dissuade me from traveling solo on my weekend adventures. One Saturday afternoon, I drove to the waterfront for shopping and lunch at Mitchell's Fish Market. It was more of a comfort for me to eat there than anything else. Mitchell's was familiar to me because there was a location right outside of the office building where I worked in Philadelphia, and seafood is my favorite dish.

It's interesting how some moments are so clear in your mind. I not only remember how satisfying it was to spend the day at the waterfront, but the service I received was so warm and friendly. The hostess saw that I was dining alone, and she brought over a newspaper for me to read and asked if she could do anything else to make me feel comfortable. I never forgot that day or that moment. It was one of the moments that made me feel good about life, even though my life was so unsettled. Four years later, I found myself at Mitchell's Fish Market in the South Hills section of Pittsburgh, but this time it was the call I received that changed the course of my life forever.

After getting married in 2008, I often teased my husband that the wining and dining went away once he put a ring on it. Ironically, we often found ourselves being entertained at some of the finest restaurants in the city, but never together. Both of our careers came with many networking and social opportunities that always involved food at a restaurant or hotel. My newly married, empty nester life was different than anything I had experienced. I was no longer a single mom chartering life on my own. I was married and living a completely different existence from the urban dwellings where I raised my children for most of our lives. I now lived in the suburban community of Mt. Lebanon, which was right outside of the city of Pittsburgh. The opposite side of the tracks, so to speak. My husband and I now spent most of our time managing our careers, caring for my mother-in-law, and forming a blended family. We traveled cross-country to visit our children, who were planted in Oregon, Arizona, and Pennsylvania.

On this Friday, a couple weeks away from the Thanksgiving holiday, I had an urge to go to Mitchell's South Hills location. This was a perfect destination for two good reasons: one, it was in the shopping mall; and two, it was only five minutes from our home.

After a long week that included several major client presentations, I was ready to relax and have a great evening with my husband. I got Atiyafied, which is my version of being glammed up for a night out on the town. Between looking marvelous and feeling the general excitement of the holiday season, I was ready for an enjoyable evening. These were the only moments that didn't evoke bad feelings toward the winter season. My anticipation was further built up by the excitement of seeing my children. The holidays were a time of large family gatherings and an opportunity to have all of us together. My daughter was away in college, my youngest son lived with his father in Maryland, and my oldest son was in Philadelphia. I missed not having my three musketeers under the same roof.

I spent so much of my life complaining about the pressures of being a single mother, often wishing that my children would grow up in an instant for this moment of freedom I now experienced. Freedom, now that I had it, wasn't all the hype I thought it would be. I missed my children immensely. The sibling fights, sticky hands, messy house, and endless noise. Although I would never advocate for single motherhood and definitely not teenage motherhood, I loved my little creatures and couldn't imagine life without them. But I would snap out of my empty nest pity party during a trip to the mall or grocery store. After watching mothers struggling with kids running around, throwing temper tantrums, and breaking items, my longing was quickly cured.

How I felt today was the complete opposite. I longed for my children to be young again, so I could bottle up time and only pour out small sips to keep them under my wings just a little longer. Through my many experiences, I've learned to savor the moment and be present while life is happening.

I wasn't comfortable with how my two sons were navigating life. My oldest son seemed to take quite a few wrong turns, and the course corrections never seemed to create a lasting change. Detour after detour landed him in dead-end streets and hazardous land mines.

I struggled to understand where things had gotten so far off track. Was I moving through life in such a frantic hurry that I missed the flashing warning signs? What was it with the young men in my family? Generation after generation, life for them was wrought with trials that for many ended in devastating outcomes. My brother lost his life to heroin, and another was murdered, and other friends and family were surely not making it out of this life alive. Diante, my youngest son, had struggled with the move to Pittsburgh. He was ten years old when we relocated and I thought he would be the one who would have the least difficulty adjusting.

At the end of the summer prior to his senior year of high school, Diante begged to leave Pittsburgh. We moved into my husband's home after I got married in 2008. Diante was leaving the friendships and community we had lived in for four years. This wasn't an easy adjustment. The thirty-minute commute between the two suburban neighborhoods caused a great divide and prevented my son from spending time with his friends. When Diante's summer vacation in Philadelphia ended, he phoned to say he was not returning home. For him, he'd rather figure out life as a runaway than return to a place to which he had never adapted. I didn't take his stance seriously at first but when I found myself explaining to him that I'd have to report him as a runaway, I knew that this was happening. I rallied my family to help talk some sense into Diante, but he managed to weasel his way out of their reach by staying with friends.

Although I eventually grew out of my love for insects, I still loved animals; just not those creepy crawlers. The tiny, scary looking bugs I once held in my hands were now considered sworn enemies. Because of this I'd never thought I would thank a spider for being the reason my son returned home. It was the poisonous bite of a brown spider that forced Diante to return to Pittsburgh for medical care. It was obvious when I got the phone call he was in despair. He'd been sleeping on a friend's couch and awoke with swelling in his upper thigh. His leg was painful and it was becoming harder to walk. We had no clue what was causing the swelling and discomfort.

The nurse in me used this medical emergency to my advantage. I informed my son that since we didn't know what was causing this problem, he needed to seek medical treatment immediately and he surely didn't want to be in the position to lose his leg. The issue with coercive tactics like this, is that sometimes those innocent "mommy" threats could become reality. My son was placed on oral antibiotics by his primary care physician. Within twenty-four hours, his conditioned worsened. He was admitted to the hospital and placed on IV antibiotics. It was determined that the bite was from a brown spider. That little creature created havoc for Diante. He was hospitalized for a week, required two surgeries, diagnosed with Methicillin Resistant Staphylococcus Aureus (MRSA), and was at risk for losing his leg. After Diante's recovery, I made the decision that his emotional health was far more important than making him stay in a place he had no desire to be in. Although it was painful to let him go to live with his father, I had to make a choice based on what he needed to grow whole and intact instead of focusing on what *I* needed, to hover and protect.

My daughter, the baby genius as I call her, was driven and determined to pursue a degree in biochemistry. She gave me a sense of comfort that at least her path was more defined, structured, and safe. Life wasn't perfect for her either though. Instead of living life out loud, she would retreat into her own quiet, safe space. I knew she was battling her own wars, but it was something about her resolve and strength that made me feel like she was going to warrior her way through.

But my oldest son, Hakeem, was the one who kept me up at night. He was the one that made me pause when I saw an unknown Philadelphia area code pop up on my phone. He was the one who seemed to keep taking the wrong turns. I wasn't comfortable with his place in life. I was filled with fear of losing him to a dark world. It was just the four of us for so much of our lives. No matter how good or bad, we always had each other and that's how I wanted life to be. The four of us plus the family that we were now united with.

For Better or Worse

MORE THAN TWENTY FAMILY MEMBERS AND FRIENDS attended our wedding at Secrets Capri Resort in Riviera Maya, Mexico. The resort did an amazing job of making this moment one of the best memories of my life. The beautiful blue skies were painted with pure, bright sunshine. The beach and ocean served as nature's perfect backdrop. Although it was the dreaded heat of August, a cool breeze enveloped the air on our special day. It was more than just bearable, it was perfect! This was God's picture-perfect canvas.

I said extra special prayers of gratitude since I feared my guests—although on the resort—wouldn't be present to experience the beauty of the wedding. It was brutally hot the day before our wedding. My husband, Mr. Perfectionist, wouldn't end the rehearsal until we all got it right. It wouldn't have been so unbearable if the ninety-plus degree weather wasn't draining the life out of us. I was the bride, but my husband was the one playing the role of Groomzilla. When I stared into the eyes of my guests, who were trying their best to hold it together, I knew it was time for me to step in. I approached my husband with a kind heart, but I needed to get the message across that we were dying out here. After what I thought was a reasonable inquiry as to when we could end the pain of rehearsal, my husband looked me straight in the eyes and asked, "Now don't you want the perfect wedding?"

"Yes," I replied. But I explained I did not want it at the expense of not having any guests show up for the real thing. Tim didn't agree with me one hundred percent, but he compromised by only making us do one more walk-through. The consolation prize was that we were at an all-inclusive resort, and refreshing frozen drinks and the choice of a pool, beach, or a room to collapse in would be our reward. My wedding was indeed perfect. Every aspect flowed just as we planned it, and the sun decided to give us a break. Life couldn't have blessed me with a better memory. Although there was trouble brewing back home in the real world, I tried my best to be present in what filled my heart with a promise for a brighter future.

There are moments in your life that literally take your breath away. For some, these moments are exhilarating and filled with excitement and anticipation, while others feel as though someone has gut-punched you, leaving you grabbing for air. Keep breathing and you'll experience both. It is human nature to want to avoid the "bad" experiences at all costs. But the reality of these experiences, whether happening around us or to us, is an inescapable one. We can't escape the complexity of life's experiences, but our responses to them and how we use them will help define our path. When life dealt the hardest gut-punch, I had to figure my way through murky waters. I could barely breathe, and part of me didn't have the desire. This journey kept teaching me the lesson of the power of choice. Choice in how I responded in a way that restored even the scarred, hardened-over areas of my heart. I had to learn that a broken heart still beats.

After just three months of marriage, we experienced what it meant when we uttered those famous words: "for better or for worse." It's amazing how quickly your life can change in what feels like the blink of an eye.

If Sorrow Comes Tomorrow

THERE ARE SOME JOURNEYS IN LIFE THAT ONE CANNOT fully relate to unless they've taken a similar path. No one's path or response to that path is the same. We are complex creatures, and although we may have the same type of experience, how we choose to respond is based on the complexities that make up our lives.

I experienced the loss of my brother, Moswen, to a heroin overdose at the young age of twenty. It was my first encounter with unimaginable pain. He was my baby brother. We planned our days around Kung-Fu flicks and old horror movies starring Dracula, Dr. Frankenstein, and the Creature from the Black Lagoon. We were inseparable. I would suck my thumb and play with his ear at the same time. My brother wasn't a thumb-sucker, but for the sake of being like his big sister, he'd put his thumb in his mouth while we played with each other's ears. Mentally gifted, baby genius, poet, and extreme introvert, my brother tried to escape the pain of this life by becoming numb to it. Losing him was devastating. Watching my mother journey through the loss was even harder.

Words are not adequate to describe the most crushing, painful heartache a parent could journey through: the loss of a child. There's an overwhelming emotional grief that manifests itself in the physical. If breathing weren't an automatic bodily response to preservation, losing a child could potentially stop your body from taking another breath. Although no one has physically assaulted you, you feel the impact of a gut punch that knocks the wind out of you and sends you doubling over. The guilt of your survival and your child's death makes you question your very existence. You don't know how it could ever be possible to go on.

It goes against the parental mindset. Losing a parent is hard too, but for a parent, you have this logical expectation that your children will bury you. There's a longing for your children to have a better and brighter future. Throughout the trials of teenage motherhood, the thought that my children would have a better existence was my fuel to never give up. Teenage motherhood didn't crush me and health conditions didn't kill me, but I was now faced with a trauma to the soul, one I didn't think I could ever recover from. Not a full recovery nor a partial recovery. I felt broken beyond repair.

I felt like I had already conquered the worst in the world. I recall so clearly not feeling defeated when my caseworker looked me straight in the eyes and said, "Three strikes, you're out." He went on to tell me that it was too hard with three children to take on the strenuous work of nursing school. "Just collect a check and stay home," he said. I could show him better than I could tell him, so I picked up my weekly bus pass and childcare subsidy and kept it moving.

I didn't wave the white flag of surrender when diabetes, high blood pressure, and kidney disease threatened my very existence. I had no intention of giving up on my son, a beautiful but troubled soul. Keemy was going to make it through the darkness. That was my hope, that's what I was fighting for.

Only a few days had passed since the November morning I had spoken with him. I was in the office meeting with one of my team members when my cell phone rang. It was important for me to know what was going on his life so ignoring his call wasn't an option. I needed to make sure he was okay. I looked at the always smiling face of my team member and asked if she'd excuse me for a second while I answered the phone.

My heart stopped racing when the tone of the conversation didn't signal an emergency. In fact, Keemy called to give me an update on how he was doing and to ask for help to pay his cell phone bill.

"Mom, I just need you to put money in my Citizens bank account," he said. "Oh, and while you're at it, can you deposit money to buy me a pair of Timbs?" he added.

"Keemy, you're pushing it. You get the boots, and I'll pay the cell phone bill," I responded with one of those laughs that contained joy and relief. He was doing okay and that was more than enough to make me smile.

Before we hung up I asked where he'd like to spend Thanksgiving. I was looking forward to making the turnpike journey to Philly. Philadelphia was home, although it wasn't the best city for young, black men. I was haunted by what was happening to them. Incarceration or death became an everyday reality. I wish the city of brotherly love lived up to its name. Keemy and I ended the call with our usual greetings: "I love you, Mom," and, "I love you, baby boy."

If sorrow comes tomorrow, I have already loved a lifetime today. The words I recited in my vows were a lie. Sorrow came in a way that crushed my soul. I replayed the events of this exchange with son. I am most grateful for his voice and the smile I felt through the phone. I am thankful that I answered it that day, because "I love you, baby boy," were the last words I spoke to Keemy. And "I love you, Mom," were the last words he spoke to me.

Two days later, my son was killed while committing a crime. I couldn't wrap my head around what transpired, and watching the news report was painful. He was on the right track, at least that's what I thought. He sold oils and other items with the other Muslim men in downtown Philly. He would often run into family members, and they would tell me how great he looked, still with that same beautiful smile plastered on his face since he was a toddler.

I later learned how he would show up at the stand where he sold oils and buy cups of coffee for the homeless guys that hung around the same downtown corner. Keemy's smile was bright, his life was turning around, and I was encouraged that we would both be all right.

There are still so many unanswered questions. After hiring a private investigator, I had to settle on the answers I did have. There's one thing to lose a child, which is a trauma in and of itself. When you add the circumstance around the death, there is another layer of pain that makes the load way too heavy to carry.

Hakeem was Keemy to us. A nickname given at birth, Keemy was a curious, full-of-life kind of child. His mischievous endeavors were brought to life through his smile. We would see that smile on his face and ask, "Keemy, what did you do?" He loved playing different sports, but football was his favorite. He started playing football in the midget league at the age of six. By the time he got to high school, his hands showed signs of a life filled with the love of the game. His fingers were disfigured, and he often complained of pain, but his love of the game never ended. I don't exactly recall when his smile started to dissipate. Keemy started getting into trouble, and was fighting at school and in the neighborhood. Counseling, family interventions, and trying to force him to church or the mosque were an uphill battle. I didn't care what spiritual path he chose, I was much more concerned that he was anchored by some kind of path at all.

There were times when we thought he was out of the woods. But, something in the streets kept pulling him back. I recalled having a serious conversation about changing his direction for good. Keemy had asked, "Mom, why do we do wrong when we know right?" That question made me think of when my mom would say, "Just because you know better, doesn't mean you do better." My family and I tried over and over to help Keemy, hoping he wouldn't bump his head too hard, as my mom would often say. She was worried that he would bump it and not return.

Our worst concern came true.

Forgiveness is Freedom

STOP REHEARSING THE PAIN. I HAD TO CONSTANTLY FEED myself that message. Rehearsing the pain is a self-inflicted act of trauma. The antidote comes in the form of forgiveness for yourself and others. Just a day after my son was killed, my sister Samira found herself standing outside of the business he was killed in front of. She said she had to be in the last place her nephew was alive. The owner came out and asked if he could help her. My sister responded, "You killed my nephew." Samira doesn't recall if she or the shop owner extended the invitation for the family to join her, but we soon appeared at the same spot where my son's chance at a different life ended.

There are parts of life during which you know without a shadow of a doubt that God's strength is what's keeping you. I know this meeting was orchestrated by God's touch. I gathered the photos I brought with me for Keemy's funeral service. I needed the owner to see a different Keemy. Not the one who showed up at his shop to take something that didn't belong to him, but the Keemy that we all knew and loved. The one that was trying hard to recover from life's wounds, but just couldn't find his way out. I needed him to know that Keemy was loved and cared for, and that his mother was sorry that she couldn't prevent so many lives from being shattered. We each showed up to express what his loss represented and how our lives would never be the same. We asked the shop owner to explain his version of the events. We asked him the same questions over and over as if we could come up with a solution to change the outcome. There was nothing he could say that would bring my son back. Although I asked why he had to shoot my son in the head, it didn't matter because that's the choice he made and I was powerless to do anything about it. I don't recall what his answer was. My mind has created its own survival tactics; not remembering all the details is one of them.

At the end of this blurry exchange, I asked if we could end our time together in prayer. I wanted to pray for forgiveness to invade our spirits, for protection from harm and evil, and for the love and peace that passeth all understanding. I held the hand of the man responsible for ending my son's life at the young age of nineteen. I held the hand of the man who ripped my heart out and crushed it into tiny pieces. I held the hand that placed one of the many thorns that occupy my side. The thorns that I will live with for the remainder of my days. I held the hands of the person that I hope will never have to be placed in a position to take someone's life ever again.

Now, I understood my mom's pain in a different way. I too, have lost a child. I found myself internalizing my mom's words: "I must continue to step through a life empty of my son." I needed God's grace to be sufficient. That would be the only way I could endure and move through the absolutely devastating and painful loss of my Keemy.

Forgiveness is a tricky thing. In my case, it was not a one-and-done act, but a circular process without an end. My mind plays tricks on me. There are days when I can't forgive myself for not being a better mom, or an older, wiser one at least, or for not having the power to save my son. There are days when I want to revoke the forgiveness extended to the person who didn't allow my son to pay for his crimes in a different way. There are days when it's hard to forgive God. Yes, I said it: forgive God for not giving my son another chance.

In my continual quest to forgive, I've learned to forgive myself for being human. God understands, more than any human being could, the act of forgiveness. Forgiveness is also required for the healing of the body. Unforgiveness is like an assault against your temple, while forgiveness carries just as much healing power as what we eat. It's nourishment at a spiritual level, removing toxicity that builds up and shows itself in physical pain and disease. I'm learning that each day is filled with an opportunity to extend the grace and forgiveness that has been extended to me.

Part II

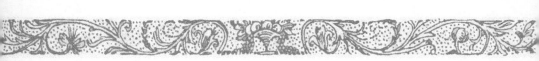

The Lessons

Lesson 1

The Journey is Not A Straight Line

MY HEALING JOURNEY ISN'T THIS PRETTY PICTURE OF doing all things in a healthy manner. Coping comes in different forms. I abused shopping and framed it as an escape from the hard work that accompanies healing. If I was going to be overweight and grief-stricken, I'd better look good from head to toe. I used to take pride in the fact that people would often say, "Atiya, I've never seen you in the same thing twice," or "Atiya, you are absolutely the best dressed!"

It became an obsessive distraction that provided a temporary escape. There was real work to be done to heal my soul. Shopping therapy wasn't it. I'll never forget the statement I made to my girlfriend Karen one year after my son's death: "I spent the kitchen." That's what I told Karen one evening as I sat on the floor in my bedroom crying and feeling utterly powerless. I emptied all the receipts from my many purses and spread them across the bedroom floor. I opened the calculator app on my cell phone and began totaling the receipts. This was my attempt to snap out of this destructive coping mechanism. I figured if I came face to face with the damage I caused through retail therapy, it would push me to find a healthier way to deal with the pain.

When Tim and I arrived home from our destination wedding, we found ourselves feverishly trying to renovate his bachelor pad into something we could both call home. Instead of getting into loan debt, we vowed to manage the home renovation project with cash. After adding up the receipts I spread across the floor, I realized that there was enough money spent to renovate the kitchen. I found myself drowning my sorrow in things that I would only wear once. I love all things fashion, but shopping in excess and accumulating things would never heal a soul in need of surgery. I had to learn this lesson repeatedly. Setting boundaries helped me to become a better financial steward of the blessings in my life. I was still going to enjoy being a fashion queen, but I would do so in a responsible manner. I often asked myself, *what am I really feeding? Pain or purpose?* One of the most important lessons I learned through grief is that the journey is not linear. You don't always graduate from one stage to the next in hopes that the pain will never surface again. The line in the healing journey is crooked, filled with twists and turns. It's rarely a straight run. I had to learn that movement through the cycles of grief was a lifelong journey. I was at peace with that revelation. It was okay to feel, to have moments, to show signs that the depth of the pain is relative to the depth of love.

I found myself apologizing or explaining why I was having a moment. Maybe it was seeing a picture of Keemy, or the anniversary of his death, or remembrance of his birth. I didn't need a reason or validation for feeling the pain of loss. People would often say, "Shouldn't you be over it by now?" We lose touch with humanity when we place a *period* where there should be a *comma*. In fact, my mom told me to stop apologizing for these moments. She said I didn't owe anyone a reason or explanation for having one, "As long as you don't stay there." That was my mom's only directive. She wanted to make sure that when I experienced a moment it was just that: a moment. Don't take up residence in the moment, and don't allow it to cause a lifetime of woes.

I learned that if I'm having a moment, getting into my car to head to the shopping mall was not the answer. It was never going to be the answer. The answer required a deeper introspective process that didn't involve the mind-numbing, instant gratification fix. Growth requires us to get ahead of it, to start foreshadowing the pain. That heightened sense of self-awareness is what's required to do something different, something healthy, something that won't come with a pile of receipts spread across the floor. It requires work, enough that has you walking forward; even if the line gets a little crooked, you know you won't be journeying backward.

Lesson 2

What's Love Got to Do with It? Everything

I AM A SURVIVOR OF AN ABUSIVE AND TOXIC RELATIONSHIP. It had such a stronghold over my life. I felt like my body was crumbling from the inside out. The dysfunction became such a part of me that leaving it for good never seemed to work out for long. I would go a month or two, or even longer, but history continued to repeat itself. My attempt to escape was like the quick fixes we find on the front of tabloid magazines. Take this magic pill to lose fifty pounds in fourteen days. Like these quick fixes touted as miracles, my attempt to leave this relationship was also an unsustainable approach that yielded results only lasting a breath or two.

Unfortunately, even the sustainable, "doable" approaches stood no chance against the rush of toxicity that coursed through my veins. This relationship could be summed up by Tina Turner's song, "What's Love Got to Do With It." The abuse became much easier to live with than the hard work required to change my life. At rock-bottom moments, I would ask myself, *is my life worth saving? And if it is, why am I allowing this relationship to kill me?* Other times, I would accept that it might just be meant for me to live like this. *But, how could anyone call this living? And why was it so hard to leave for good? Why am I not making different choices?* These questions ran through my mind dozens of times.

It wasn't that I didn't know what the right choices were. It was just that the bad choices felt better. Even if the feeling was temporary. My abuser was so convincing that it wouldn't hurt. *Go for it. Everybody else is doing it.* Although the temptations were everywhere, a way out was always present. These fork-in-the-road moments were wrought with anxiety. Yes, there was an escape route, but it was so hard to break the cycle. I knew I was the only one who could save my life. No one could do this for me. I don't care how many resources or helping hands were out there; ultimately, the choice had to be mine. The power was in my hands to choose life, and I had to become sick and tired of being sick and tired. I had to stand up strong and come face to face with my abuser. The same strength and courage my mom possessed was passed down to me. Rock-bottom came and staying was no longer an option. It was time for a confrontation and I knew that only one of us would survive it.

My abuser was *me*, and the weapon I used to harm my body was *food*! It was purely a love-hate relationship. I loved everything about my favorite foods. The taste, texture, look, and smell. Food evoked memories of good times with family, outings with friends, and great moments with the kids. We all have foods that we can't deny. Mine are served at every holiday meal. When both sides of the family can burn, the abuse is almost inescapable. There's not a dish cooked by my family that I don't like. You name it, and I've tried it and liked it: macaroni and cheese, sweet potatoes, collard greens, string beans, potato salad, turkey with stuffing, and don't forget the gravy. Add fresh dinner rolls, and the list goes on and on. I can go without dessert, but please don't deny me the rest of the forbidden carbs. Just let me eat and succumb to a couch coma and I promise to stay put for the remainder of the day. Actually, I had no other choice but to stay put. My body's resources were in slug mode, held captive until it recovered from the heavy load I placed on it. It's okay to indulge occasionally, but I started making everyday a special occasion and that was not working for me, and definitely not for my health.

Single motherhood had me making good excuses daily. Night shift nursing, school activities, and a host of other competing priorities were all legitimate reasons why the quick and easy meals were the answer. I was tired and overworked. How could I possibly make healthier food choices when I'm in a constant battle with time and energy? The boxed hamburger helper only takes a few ingredients and one pot. The boxed macaroni and cheese has everything in it. Boil the macaroni, use the fake cheese, and voilà, dinner is served. We could eat cereal for any meal, and lunchmeat sandwiches on potato bread were the best. My lack of time excuse was convincing and easily solved by the ready-made, food-like substances found up and down the middle aisles of grocery stores. Pick up any box, read the label, and try pronouncing the ingredients. Better yet, look at the expiration date. Does it last for a year?

I made these choices so easily, justifying the fact that I would supplement the meal with vegetables. Day in, day out, the quick fixes became a staple. Lunchboxes were filled with the infamous Lunchables, juice in a box, and topped off with a piece of fruit. We ate healthy foods, but not nearly enough for our bodies to get about the business of functioning properly and healing itself. Knowing better isn't doing better. Application is the only way to change your future. I knew better, and now I needed to do better. When everything else was hard, it was easy to take shortcuts on some of the most important aspects of living a healthy life. I got so caught up with life that it became so easy to ignore the damage I was creating on the inside. We often get caught up in trying to get away with something. We think if no one sees us, then it's okay. We sneak food and try to hide our addictions. But while we're trying to fool others, the only thing we're accomplishing is hurting ourselves. Spanx, one pill wonders, magic creams, and numerous get-fit-quick schemes have helped us run from the nothing that chases. Trust me, I've indulged in them all enough to know firsthand. These quick fixes helped me manage my time by spending it doing other things on the endless mommy-do-list.

What is it that you're holding on to for dear life? What is it that you choose to not let go of because the hurt feels so good? When the rush fizzles out, when the abuse takes our life, when the money is gone, what are we left with? False Evidence Appearing Real—FEAR—that made us believe we needed that crap in the first place.

My awakening process didn't happen overnight. As a survivor of domestic violence, I know that the journey is not as easy as what folks on the outside believe it is. I am still struggling, still falling. The only difference between now and then is that I choose to live life more conscious of how my actions either deposit life or deposit death into my spirit. I won't allow another human being to inflict harm on my life and that includes me. Now, when I decide something that's not aligned with what feeds my mind, body, and spirit in a positive way, I get in touch with the emotional state I'm in and seek to understand the fix I'm really seeking. What hurts, and/or what am I afraid of? With each decision that takes me away from saving my life, I realize that running from nothing is just as irrational as it sounds. Ultimately the unhealthy choices are not worth dying for. So what's love got to do with it? Everything!

Lesson 3

Build-A-Body

ALL EYES WERE ON ME AS I WALKED INTO A ROOM FILLED with men and women in their evening's best dress. Everyone was having a great time enjoying the festivities the evening prior to Fun, Fit & Fabulous women's health conference. I looked good and felt great. Earlier that day, my husband and I spent the afternoon driving from Pittsburgh, Pennsylvania to Charleston, West Virginia for the annual conference. It was a picture-perfect fall day filled with the beautiful scenery of colors, tree-covered mountains, and sunshine guiding our way. Except for the bank calling to ask if I was in Connecticut, shopping at Target, all was well in our world. Apparently, you can create fake debit cards and go on shopping sprees. Thank goodness for the folks at the bank who, after the first time I fell prey to an attack, made sure I was always kept on alert. The unfortunate part was that the bank had to shut my debit card down. The fortunate part was that I got to spend my husband's money for the weekend.

I loved the dress I wore to the reception. A black, off the shoulder, jewel-encrusted, swing dress. It was a hit, but the accessories underneath became the main topic of the evening. Who would have thought a compliment on how I looked would spark a conversation that had the women high-fiving and nearly falling out of our chairs in laughter? We each shared the joys and struggles of womanhood, especially the amount of energy it took to look good. Outfits, especially for special events, are planned all the way down to what we'll wear to hold in the undesirable parts. The pursuit of building the perfect body took me down memory lane to Build-A-Bear, a place in malls across America that allows little kids and adults to build a teddy bear made by your own hands.

My kids and I have always gotten a kick out of going to Build-A-Bear. We didn't go often, simply because you needed a small fortune by the time you added all the parts, clothing, and accessories. At Build-A-Bear, you control the entire process of creating your new buddy. You get to stuff it, dress it, and place a heart inside. You can also make it laugh, just like the one I made in memory of my son Keemy. The best part about Build-A-Bear is that you leave with something that was created by you. Just like Build-A-Bear, there are some fashion tricks that have allowed women to build our bodies, if only for one night.

I don't how it happened, but during the Fun, Fit & Fabulous reception, the ladies found themselves at the table talking freely about everything. We didn't have to censor our conversation since the men were off entertaining themselves. Compliments circled the table about lipstick colors, hairstyles, and dresses. Our compliments toward one another sparked a conversation around the secrets of building the best body, no exercise or diets needed. Yes, we get caught up in the traps of industries targeting women to believe they have the answer to helping us build a perfect body. From Spanx to Jockey, I had it all. These undergarments cost as much the dress. I couldn't live without them because the smooth, shapely silhouette they helped build proved to be well worth the investment. These fashion must-haves become our besties. They help pull it all together, tight and right, if only for one night.

I began to share my Build-A-Body secrets that had us whispering, giggling, and acting like little girls playing with Barbie and Ken dolls. There are fashion undergarments that can give you a boob or butt job, annihilate the muffin top, reverse the thunder thighs, and smooth out the caterpillar back. I have so many of these items they have their own dedicated dresser. It doesn't matter what you're wearing; there's an undergarment made to fit all types of attire, including short dresses, long dresses, off the shoulder, or strapless. The secret of how great I looked was in the carefully chosen fashion undergarments. These wardrobe enhancements can sometimes feel like a contraption that may require assembly assistance. Just ask my husband.

Now, there are some rules you should follow when determining which fashion undergarment to use. For one, the butt enhancer is one that requires the most discretion. This undergarment is for those who desire a little more junk in their trunk, but don't want to spend a fortune, die trying, risk a plastic surgery faux pas, or put in enough time doing the tried-and-true glute builders. The key is to pay close attention to the tips, tricks, and traps of this wardrobe addition. You'll also have to find one that's realistic enough that you don't feel like you've added water balloons or even worse—an over-inflated basketball under your dress.

Once you find the perfect one, you'll need to decide when and where to wear it. The first time is always scary, and for those of you who feel a little nervous about wearing the butt enhancer I suggest you try out your new addition on vacation. This will hopefully protect your anonymity. Now, if you run into your pastor or spiritual leader on vacation or anyone else that knows that there's no way on Earth you were blessed that way, please try not to turn around and walk away. That just might create more problems. Hello!

The first time I wore this figure enhancer was to a black-tie gala. I had on a fabulous brushed silver halter mermaid dress. My attempt at secretly slipping the undergarment on was a failure. As soon as I turned around my husband asked, "Is there something you want to talk about?" My response was no. This conversation soon became a full-blown confession of my desire to add some jelly to my jam. Well, that lame excuse wasn't satisfactory enough. My husband flatters me no matter what. Skinny or thick, it doesn't matter to him. I'm perfect just the way I am. There was no need to create the illusion of what I think is the perfect body because his attraction to me is not superficial. It was me that had a problem with my body. The extra tire layers I carried around my middle would have been better placed on my rear. The butt enhancer was a futile attempt at creating a better proportioned physique. I spent years wondering why I wasn't blessed with a booty like my older sister, Samira, only to find out that she often wondered why she didn't have my boobs. Isn't that what we all do? Highlight our imperfections and covet what others have.

I created my own Build-A-Body workshop in my wardrobe. I stuffed some places while lifting and tightening others. My attempt at building the perfect body was far more expensive than stuffing a bear at the local mall. It not only cost a fortune for these wardrobe enhancements, but also wearing them came at the expense of not being able to eat or breathe—two essential components of staying alive. I often forfeited comfort to look good in my own skin. The temporary fix was good for a night. Once the tightening and lifting game was over, things fell apart in the privacy of my home.

Getting up and repeating the same routine was exhausting. And let's not even talk about what happened in the summertime. It can be ninety degrees at a summer wedding and not only do you have to contend with breathing and eating issues, you should add susceptibility to heat stroke. The wardrobe enhancements became more like wardrobe hell.

I was aware that a wardrobe full of contraptions worn to create the illusion of a perfect body wasn't the right journey to save my life. I was still the same person struggling with a healthy body image. I wanted to look in the mirror at a more aesthetically pleasing physique and knock a few medications out of my ever-growing pill box. The superficial enhancements would never get me to the *me* I so desired to be.

In the safe confines of my home, the many masks were removed and I still had to deal with the person that most people didn't get to see in public. All the undergarments and the beautiful wardrobe that garnered much attention wouldn't change the work that needed to occur for me to live my best life. Each night I repeated the same routine of taking them off, washing them, and placing them back in a drawer. Looking in the mirror was an inescapable way of facing what remained.

If I was so sick and tired of being sick and tired, then why couldn't I change for good? Some say it's not rocket science. But, it sure feels like it. I understood that behavior change is one of the most difficult aspects of any type of course correction. It is not easy trying to shed ingrained behaviors, let alone fighting against the giants of a health-hostile world. I needed my heart and mind to get on the same page. I had to be relentless in my approach.

I sometimes laughed at all the wardrobe enhancements available to help build a body. But, I know that some enhancements are not a laughing matter. Women are being severely disfigured and losing their lives after trying to build a body through plastic surgery.

This Build-A-Body workshop we find ourselves in is not a joking matter. Going as far as seeking illegal ways to get a bigger booty causes a lot of harm, both physically and financially. The photos of the destruction are enough to bring you to tears. Mothers, wives, daughters, and sisters are not returning home because their search for a better body caused them to pay the ultimate price with their lives.

Every social media channel is an advertisement for a basketball booty and water balloon boobies. The photos posted aren't showing off other beautiful features, such as a woman's eyes or her smile. The display is all focused on showing off assets that get the most attention from people that don't even deserve to look. That true, deep down, I-love-you-no-matter-what beauty comes from honoring our temples and being grateful for the skin we're in.

I needed a new heart, and not the plastic, red object used in stuffing a Build-A-Bear. I needed a real one with a strong beat that would give me the perseverance and courage to change my body for good. Saving my life was going to require changing my heart. It's not how I look that makes me healthy; it's how I live. My heart is real. Our hearts are real. They beat with a knowing that we are enough.

I was trying to build the facade of a perfect physique that I could only call my own for a few hours. If only for one night, I looked perfect under that beautiful brushed silver mermaid dress. I had the body I dreamed of, diet and exercise not required. For me to be liked or accepted, I needed to create an illusion of Atiya that was good enough for the world. I wanted that good feeling to last longer than one night. For that to happen, I had to love myself so much that I was willing to get on the path to the ideal body that required real work. Work that is sometimes hard and tiring, but work that would produce results that I didn't have to put back in a drawer at the end of the night.

Marilyn Monroe was spot-on when she said that women are measured by their numbers and shapes. Does she have the perfect physique: 36-24-36? Is she round in the right places? Marilyn desired for herself, and all women, to be measured for what really counted: the person she was becoming on the inside.

I never wore the butt enhancer after that night. It was a perpetrator that would never give me the permanent feeling of what living healthily was all about. If I wanted to see any part of my body change, the change would come by building my best body through the healthy choices I made. My Build-A-Body workshop would include real body parts, no artificial fillers or preservatives added. It would be a workshop deserving of a lifetime commitment.

Lesson 4

Everyone Needs a Karen

I WASN'T MY NORMAL CHATTY SELF AS MY HUSBAND AND I drove to work. Usually, once I get talking, it takes a subtle tap or some other hint from Tim that I need to be quiet or at least take a breath between sentences.

I was filled with nervous energy that morning. I had already concluded that what I was about to share was going to be met with resistance. I was even more concerned that Tim would finally think I had gone off the deep end. I thought that at least if I shared the news during our morning commute, I would have an eight-hour workday to escape Tim's interrogation about my bright idea.

"I've decided to run the Pittsburgh half marathon," I blurted out as if saying it fast would make his reaction any less painful. Based on the side-eyed look Tim gave me, maybe sharing this news in the car, while he was driving, wasn't such a good idea after all. I needed Tim to keep his eyes on the road and hands on the steering wheel instead of whipping his neck around to say, "You can't run a half marathon."

It didn't take Tim long to share with me just how daunting this new challenge would be. He explained that running a half marathon would be like leaving home, running to my office, running back home, and then running halfway back to the office. Well, when he put it that way I thought to myself, *he's probably right. There's no way I could run a half marathon.*

It took a minute for me to process this news since I hadn't calculated exactly what a half marathon really meant. I found myself visualizing running from home and back, not once, but several times. Despite hearing such daunting news, the strength in me responded differently.

Running the half marathon was another step of demonstrating I could do hard things. It would symbolize my courage to stand up to the impossibilities of life. Yes, I too thought I must have lost my mind. I was not a runner, and did not find enjoyment in running. The fact that my husband knew this about me didn't help my plight. The good news was that no matter how ridiculous the idea sounded to my husband, I was already set on running. Usually, when I get to the point of sharing my bright ideas with Tim, my decision has already been made. I just think it would be polite if he knew about it.

My husband is my champion and his way of caring is through protecting me. Tim's concerns were valid. Having diabetes, high blood pressure, and kidney disease signaled in his mind: *she's too sick to be doing this. She's not a runner, her knees are bad, and it's a half marathon, for crying out loud.* I knew exactly what was running through his mind because, although I hated to admit it, these thoughts were also running through mine.

I shared my impossible half marathon adventure with my girlfriend Karen, who, unlike my husband, was supportive from the jump. "Well, if you're going to run for Keemy, I'm going to be right alongside you," she said. I'm telling you: girlfriends should be a part of every marriage contract. When your husband doesn't get it, your girlfriends will. Girlfriends are your co-conspirators; they push you, cheer for you, and encourage you to never quit your daydream. They help you conquer the most difficult challenges, especially the ones that seem impossible to overcome.

Four years had passed since my son's death. Instead of allowing the date of his death, his birthdate, and all the other significant milestones to be filled with a cloud of grief, the marathon would be a healthy detour, something to look forward to, something aspirational to hold onto. A memory filled with triumph rather than despair. I visualized my son smiling and saying, "Mom, you have to keep moving." Yes, I was still moving for him, for me. And I was going to do what he was no longer able to: live.

During my half marathon training, friends, colleagues, and even strangers overwhelmed me with encouragement. Not one person said a word about the impossibilities of this journey. They didn't express any notion about me being an inexperienced, non-runner with multiple chronic conditions setting forth on mission impossible.

They were encouragers like Marnie, an accomplished runner who didn't take my journey lightly. Marnie, who wears sensible shoes, didn't dismiss me, the glamour chick who wore five-inch heels' desire to run the half-marathon. Instead, she listened intently as I expressed my fears. Marnie didn't encourage me to do something else or something less strenuous to honor my son's memory. She instead used the power of her tongue to light a fire so bright within my soul. A fire that screamed that I was going to accomplish what I set out to do, run my first half marathon.

> **Marnie:** *I was thinking more about you doing the half marathon and I realized another reason why you will do it, and do it well. You will find yourself surrounded by thousands of other people who, for one reason or another, have decided to do something that to others seems crazy. Every runner there has a story. They are running to honor the memory of their son. They are running to prove to themselves that they can do what seems un-do-able. They are running because they desperately miss someone who passed away from cancer and know that no matter how much pain they may feel while they run or walk, they will not outrun the pain of missing the person they lost. But they will honor the struggle that person made to live life and pass on with as much dignity and grace as they could muster.*

These are the stories you will think about as you pass people and as you get passed. You will smile at strangers that you will never see again and sometimes give them encouragement. You will have strangers staring at you in amazement as you walk or run down the road and they will see your bib and they will cheer for you and your story. That's what you need to think about when you think of doing the race. Don't think of 13 miles. Thirteen miles is nothing compared to the stories you have lived and the stories others have lived. Think of the web of stories that will be swirling around you as you run down the road. It is a wonderful feeling to think of collective struggle of which you will be a part. Just breathe and smile. Breathe in peace and smile out support. Isn't that really just about the only and best thing we can all do in our everyday lives anyway? Enjoy the whole experience. Enjoy the cheers and the smiles and the craziness of it all. Carry your son with you and know that it is a great thing you are doing.

This quote by Cicely Tyson, posted in my cubicle, helps me. Challenges make you discover things about yourself that you never really knew. They're what make the instrument stretch— what make you go beyond the norm."

Marnie's words didn't lay dormant in an email. I deposited every word into my heart. On May 4, 2012, my half marathon bib read "Run4MYSON" and when our legs gave out, Karen and I finished the race with our hearts.

We're all facing a myriad of challenges. They are inescapable and just as much a part of our life as breathing. The power is always in our response. My ability to bounce back was strengthened by the bonds of family, friendship, and even strangers with whom I may never cross paths again. When my optimism dips, I have a circle surrounding me, helping me get up, and refusing to allow me to wallow in defeat. They are the secret ingredients to believing that I always have a choice as to how I show up. They help me see life through different perspectives. They sometimes join in the pity party but only to help me turn it into a victory party. We were designed to thrive off connectedness. Not just any kinds of connections, but connections with people who will help you defeat the giants. People who bring an energy, a faith walk that inspires you to believe that you are possible!

Lesson 5

Slow Down and Breathe

WE LIVE IN SUCH A FRANTIC STATE OF EXISTENCE. SLOWING down and simply being conscious of our breath is a delicacy that we don't indulge in enough. I too am guilty of this lifestyle. There were times I would get a frantic phone call from my youngest son's school asking me to come up immediately. "He's out of control again!" Thank goodness I lived and worked in our neighborhood so no destination was more than a few blocks away. I'd arrived at his school ready to snatch him out of class and give him an old-fashioned one. Instead, since I just left a labor and delivery unit helping a woman in labor breathe through the pain, I thought I'd try it on him. "Breathe, Diante, breathe," I said. If deep breathing can help a woman bringing life into the world, it could surely help this second grader get his life right.

If I had it my way, every person who must drive in rush hour would be required to take deep breathing classes. Rush hour is a period where people transform into talking Medusa heads. Once we became empty nesters, Tim and I made a lifestyle change. We wanted to escape the unbearable morning and evening rush hour madness. Moving into the city was the best decision for my healthy journey.

We found an 1850s Victorian home located in the Mexican War Streets, a section of Pittsburgh's Northside community. Everything about this move was good for my health. I walked to work—except during winter because we just don't get along—lived near a park with a man-made lake, had neighbors that became friends, and avoided rush hour madness. I was done with the experience of the bewitching hour. Our Medusa personalities are witnessed through glass windows as people engage in full-blown screaming matches with other drivers who can't even hear a word they're saying. Evil eyes, shouting expletives, and a blaring horn concerto are evidence that I'm not alone in the self-regulation and shallow breath department.

Now, this isn't all about judgment and I have not turned into a poster-child of "Peace be upon you." There are no innocent parties when it comes to this, and if I'm honest with you, I too am a recovering Medusa head. I've experienced one too many embarrassing moments when Medusa took over my innocent body and forced me to behave in a way that was not admirable.

On one particularly sunny day, I became trapped in what felt like a parking lot on the street. I couldn't understand what could possibly be holding us hostage. It was five o'clock, so I originally chalked it up to typical rush hour traffic. It didn't take long for the yelling to ensue, the horn symphony to begin, and our downright impatient nature to invade our bodies.

At this point in my life, I'd had learned the hard way to stay calm, breathe, and stop sweating stuff you have no control over. I mean, was I going to get out of my car, pick up every car in front of me, and move them to the side so I can proceed? No. So, on this day while I was on my best behavior, I didn't mind pulling over to put my convertible top down and wait patiently until traffic started moving again. As the traffic story unfolded, I found out that my rush hour conclusion wasn't the total cause of the parking lot conditions. To my surprise, there was more to this traffic story. It wasn't just rush hour that was holding us up.

When I put the top down, my view became unobstructed. My heart was lightened, taking in the scene. Closer to the traffic light was a family of geese trying to make their way across the street. There were two adult geese and what looked like at least a half-dozen baby geese. They weren't alone. They had traffic angels in the form of three people who created a safe passage by blocking the cars from proceeding. These beautiful ones served as a barrier between the geese and the angry drivers. The distance between where the geese were and the river where they would be safe was short. However, the path was dangerous. You see, the angry drivers' limited view caused them to get caught up in their own world. They could only see the constant cycle of the lights turning green, then yellow, then red without any traffic movement.

Pulling over to the side to put my top down provided me with a vision of the activity at the light. My journey to get home immediately turned from me to them. I felt the shift in my energy and all that mattered in that moment was their safety. My disposition changed because of the evidence before me. I could only imagine how frightened the geese were with all the blaring of horns and people yelling out of their windows. I could only imagine the angst felt by the helpful traffic angels trying their best to herd the geese to safety. It took several minutes to finally usher the geese out of the street, but those in the back with the blocked view probably felt it was more like an hour.

We get so caught up trying to get to a destination that we can't appreciate where we are in the moment. My whole perspective changed once the vision of the geese were in focus. *How would I have reacted if this information was not revealed to me? Would I have joined the talking Medusa heads?*

I recall driving on 69th Street in Upper Darby, a section right outside of Philadelphia. I was at an intersection when a man traveling with several passengers made an abrupt turn in front of me. As I was about to have a road rage moment, I realized that the man and passengers were my Abi, grandmother, and other relatives. It would have been a hard recovery if my Abi experienced road rage inflicted by his daughter. The toxicity of our attitude and behaviors has a negative effect on the person inflicting the pain as well as the one receiving it.

Through the Integrated Medicine department at Allegheny General Hospital in Pittsburgh, a movement designed to bring health and healing in a non-traditional way is inspiring employees and patients to use their breath, among other self-management tools, to bring a sense of calm into what can be a hectic environment. After attending a half-day mind-body workshop, a technique Laura Crooks, RN and Wellness Coach, shared would have been so helpful to the dozens of people creating such a dysfunctional orchestra of sounds on that evening when a family of geese were trying to make it home. Or, to me during the encounter with my Abi. Slow, deep breaths send an immediate message to your brain to slow down and relax; all is well. Laura joked that many of her clients expressed how useful the simple art of breathing was during some heated situations, traffic being one of them.

Being the child that most resembles my mother's personality, I have a strong tendency to react before breathing. I have been known to claim being the victim of emotional hijacking. Unfortunately, my dear husband is sometimes the innocent bystander of these hijacked moments. Awareness is the first step to changing behavior, especially one that is not becoming. I hear the words, "just breathe," and I'm suddenly reminded of the responsibility to bring peace into the world through my response. STOP. That's what I learned from Deepak Chopra. STOP gives our mouth an opportunity to be slow to speak. This acronym is intended to help you gather yourself before responding. Taking deep breaths to allow your body to relax and become centered. When you observe yourself, it's as if you're looking in the mirror and whatever you were going to say if you said those same words to yourself, consider whether would it deposit life or death into your spirit. If it's the latter, then stopping allows you to redirect and proceed by extending grace and compassion.

I've had to be deliberate in making choices that would rejuvenate and heal my most damaged parts, beginning with slowing down and breathing.

Lesson 6

It's Not Worth the Pain

IT WAS 1:30 A.M., AND I WAS UP DOING MY NORMAL, DYS-functional routine of letting Nemo and Dory out in the middle of the night. Caesar, the Dog Whisperer, would surely classify me as one of "those" dog owners. I believe I trained my dogs to be paranoid about having an accident in the house. Around the same time in the middle of the night, Nemo and Dory wake me up with their normal, shake-our-bodies-as-hard-as-we-can routine.

On this night, my hands were swollen, feet were tingling, and stomach was on fire from the restaurant food I ate on Sunday night. Although broiled fish was the healthiest food on the menu, the sodium content made it feel like the fish took a bath in a bowl of salt. It's hard to fall back to sleep after my midnight routine with the dogs, but the added physical and emotional discomfort from my so-called healthy dinner made me even more miserable.

My dinner outing was the result of a deal with my husband. I paid for an item on a rare and almost non-existent shopping outing with him. Dinner was his treat.

In the days of our courtship, there was never a time I would say no to a dinner date. On this occasion, I should have spoken up about the real healthy dinner I had prepared earlier at home. Instead, I gave in to the emotional draw of going on a date with my husband. As soon as he said the words, "dinner is on me," my mind began to race as to where would we eat and what the heck would I find on the menu that wouldn't kill me.

121

The fish was broiled, but I knew from hello that the glistening golden liquid substance was not from plain water, but rather, salt on top of fat and more salt. Surely the culprits that joined the broiled fish were a combination of butter and seasonings that stripped all signs of healthy from the fish. Bloating, gas, swollen hands and feet, and emotional anguish at 1:30 a.m. overshadowed the dreamy reward of date night.

Two Alka-Seltzer chewable tablets later, the guilt syndrome set in as I replayed the decisions that led up to my misery. Food should not have been the reward for sharing the financial responsibility. To further add insult to injury is the fact that I was prepared to enjoy a healthy, healing, and guilt-free dinner at home because I took the time to prepare my meals earlier that afternoon.

My mom's wisdom usually shines through during my ah-ha moments. I could hear her voice loud and clear when she said, "When you make a decision to eat the entire pint of Haagen-Dazs ice cream, know you are making a choice. Good, bad, or indifferent, you're making a choice." Eating with a sense of awareness means taking responsibility. Pause and reflection could have resulted in my husband and me going home, enjoying a healthy dinner together, and going to bed minus the swollen hands, feet, and upset stomach.

Now, that change in course may not have prevented the usual midnight dog outing—the dog whisperer will need to help me with that one. But at least my body and mind would have rejoiced that I took one more step, one more choice for health.

Lesson 7

Eviction Notices

My husband is the glass half-full kind of guy. The smile that's plastered on his face is permanent, like the makeup you can get tattooed on your lips. His view of the world and see-the-good-in-it kind of attitude is sometimes annoying, especially when I'm in the mood to feel sorry for myself.

In July 2011, I received a message in my inbox stating my online health tracker had been updated with my latest lab results. Now, to paint the perfect picture, I always took pride in how perfect my labs had become over the course of my illnesses. I expected nothing to be out of whack.

At eleven p.m., when I should have been getting in bed to get enough sleep, I had the bright idea to check my labs. My confident, perfect lab smile changed to a frown, which turned into sobs of defeated tears. The labs that measured my kidney function showed an elevation in one of the tests. Every principle of positive thinking, stress management, and the glass half-full approach went right out the window. I gave up, cursed creation, and told my husband I was doomed.

I immediately began to create an excuse for canceling the next day's gatherings. Sobbing, closed curtains, and lying in bed all day would replace church, brunch, and fellowship with my circle of friends.

My husband, the encourager, went into full mode. He grabbed my hands and began to pray. I closed my eyes, took several deep breaths, and started to calm down until he got to the part of the prayer where he thanked God for giving my kidneys full life beyond the five years I was told I had. At that moment, I opened one eye to see him with both eyes closed. Out of my love, honor, and respect I have for my husband and my reverence for God, I stopped looking at him cock-eyed and refrained from interrupting his prayer to ask had he lost his mind. I mean, didn't he hear what I just shared with him about my labs? My kidney disease was showing signs of progression. *I'm losing the battle. How can you thank God?* I thought.

I stopped my pity party and side-eyed looks before the prayer ended, and I thanked him. I was still planning on canceling everything, but my husband's next move told me otherwise. He said, "Atiya, I get it. Your labs results are not what you hoped for, but you're not canceling anything tomorrow. You made a commitment to yourself to go to church and enjoy time with your friends at brunch. I will not leave you here to wallow in self-pity nor will I encourage you to look at this as the end."

My husband's stance was unusual. I was used to him allowing me to get my way. I prayed myself to sleep and woke up drawing up a new eviction notice for Mrs. Crooks and her rowdy kids (the name I've given my health conditions).

That morning, my eviction notice consisted of taking slow deep breaths, placing my hands on the part of my back where my kidneys reside, and thanking them for working so hard to get rid of the waste in my system. I thanked them for defying the odds. I envisioned the sun emitting its powerful rays into the darkened areas of my kidneys that prevented them from working properly. I visualized my kidneys healing themselves. Finally, I asked for forgiveness for ingesting food and substances that made it easier for Mrs. Crooks and her crew to cause damage. I put on my game face, got dressed, and went about the business of having a fabulous day! Who or what do you need to serve an eviction notice to?

Lesson 8

Be Afraid of the Dark

I MUST TELL YOU THAT THESE MOMENTS OF OVERWHELMING fear of the future enveloped me more often than I'd like to admit. When I discovered two lumps in my neck, the nurse in me jumped to the worst possible diagnosis. Several tests, including blood work and ultrasounds, revealed undesirable possibilities. Lupus was one of them!

I absolutely loved my primary care physician. Dr. Lemley was truly my partner in health. Her transparency, communication, and genuine concern made me feel like I was more than just a patient. She called me one evening while I was attending an event.

"Atiya, one of your lab results is an indication for lupus," she said.

An immediate switch went off and the noise from the crowded room became muffled and distorted. "Dr. Lemley, what did you say?" I asked. I heard her clearly the first time but couldn't bring myself to acknowledge what she said.

"Atiya, we have to conduct more tests to make a definitive diagnosis, but I wanted to share this with you. You have other elevated blood work. So, I want you to stop taking your cholesterol medications."

My festive mood immediately shifted as I ran out of the event, quickly handed over my valet ticket, and impatiently waited for my car. After I got off the phone with Dr. Lemley, I immediately started a Google search on my cell phone. I saw how lupus affected the lives of my family members. Quite frankly, I couldn't imagine having to deal with one more thing.

My pillbox fluctuated depending on how well I was doing with living a healthy lifestyle. I was tired of the constant threat of chronic conditions, and now there was yet another reason for me to be afraid. How would lupus impact my other conditions? My quality of life? My life expectancy? My ability to work and support my family? I was filled with so many questions and emotions. I called Samira and shared the news. I went home and cried on Tim's shoulders. Tim didn't know what the hell lupus was; however, from my reaction, he knew it was something that could severely alter my life—our lives.

I wanted to keep this information contained. I had no desire to put any more weight on my family. My family would freak out if I had shared this news. They worried about me so much. When they asked about me, I always answered, "I'm fine." No matter what, that's what I choose to put out in the universe.

One month later, the few family and friends with whom I shared this news were starting to ask about the additional tests. I used every excuse, including "I haven't heard from Dr. Lemley," and "the hospital hasn't released the records yet."

Truth be told, after spending so much time researching lupus and talking to my cousin about her life living with this condition, I wasn't actively seeking any additional results. I was okay living in the dark because I was afraid. Instead of facing the reality and getting about the business of confronting this battle, I retreated into the so-called safe space of ignorance.

I finally got up the nerve to reach out to Dr. Lemley to say let's move forward. If we must repeat tests, then let's do it. Waiting on the hospital system to do their job could end up harming me. That week, I received a script in the mail with a laundry list of more blood work to get done. I neatly folded the script and carried it in my purse for safekeeping.

After all that talk, I was still afraid and willing to live in the dark. I made up every excuse to delay getting the tests done. Although the blood work didn't need to be done while fasting, I convinced myself that they *must* be fasting labs. So, oops, I just drank my smoothie. I guess I'll have to get them done another day. I drank a smoothie every morning for a month.

A text message from my sister changed the game for me. You know how you can see the message without having to open it? Well, I saw her text and was trying to figure out how to avoid responding. My excuses had become lies. I knew it was time to stop. Our text conversation disclosed the fact that I had yet to get my blood work done and had been carrying around the script for more than a month:

Sis: *Did u get ur test results back?*

Me: *I didn't get them done yet. I made a commitment to get them done this week.* (lie)

Sis: *What's taking so long?*

Me: *Fear.*

Sis: *The doctor hasn't called you? You would have a cow if I did that. Knowledge is power, right???* (Throwing my words and mindset right back at me). *I understand.* (This was my sister's way of trying to be gentle, but I know she was frustrated with my lack of follow-through.)

Me: *I called her. She sent me the script for additional testing. The script is in my purse* (insert-exhaustive smiley face).

Sis: *Words you would say to me- 'I don't want to lose you.' My sister, please get the tests. It could very well be nothing. Love u.*

Me: *I know-* (insert heart) *I'm going to make a commitment to get them done tomorrow or Thursday.*

Sis: *Thank u.*

The next day, I texted Samira and told her I got my labs done. I wanted to tell her about the ordeal I had to go through to get them done.

It's not easy drawing my blood. I took the convenient route and went to the health center in my office building. Several needle sticks later, I walked over to Quest Diagnostics. I confessed that I just might have made her job harder. This phlebotomist is always so kind and professional, but it even got to her to see my arms beat up. Two more sticks, and she filled a boatload of tubes. She warned me that I was going to have a couple of nasty bruises. At that point, it didn't matter.

I was on my way to the light. I was ready to face my fears and *still* get about the business of living. I was going to share all this drama with my sister, but I was reminded of a passage I read in Deepak Chopra and Dr. Rudolph Tanzi's book, *Super Genes*. The authors wrote about "stress dumping," so I thought it best that there wasn't a need to share all the details. My sister was carrying enough. This inconvenient, minor pain-filled, bruised arm was my burden to shoulder. That was on a Wednesday.

That Friday, while catching the bus to volunteer at Bethlehem Haven women's shelter, my phone rang. It was Dr. Lemley.

"Atiya, your labs are fine," she said.

Again, as if I didn't hear her right the first time, I asked, "What do you mean?"

"Atiya, you don't have lupus. All your labs are normal and the ANA is down to a level that isn't clinically significant."

Again, instead of accepting this hallelujah praise moment, I asked, "Is there anything I need to be concerned about? What about my blood counts? What about my liver tests?"

In her most patient, but happy to share good news voice, Dr. Lemley repeated the good news. "You're fine. Have a good weekend Atiya."

I got off that bus with the biggest, makes-your-mouth-hurt smile. I don't have lupus! I wanted to apologize to all the lupus social media channels I had subscribed to. I wanted to let them know I was an imposter. I was all ready to sport my favorite color, purple, in support of lupus. I had liked so many pages in support of fighting the disease, signed up for newsletters, and practically began to live and think like I had the condition. Yes, I know what you're thinking. I am slightly off, but aren't we all to some extent?

I only had a few minutes before getting to the women's shelter, so I made a few calls and sent text messages. I walked around in the dark because of *fear* over nothing. And guess what? Even if I had the disease, I was relinquishing my power by feeding it.

When it comes to life, you can't let fear of the unknown prevent you from living, or better yet, force you into a paralytic state. I don't care if it's a diagnosis or other life change. Face it! I sent my sister a text message saying if I remembered how to skip, I would sure be doing just that, even with my broken-down knee.

The sun was shining bright, I was on my way to volunteer, and I had just received news that blessed me so. Yes, I felt like skipping. In her ever-so-supportive way, Samira encouraged me to do something else besides skip. The last thing she wanted to hear was that my victory skip turned into another trip to the surgeon. So, with her advice, I took a walk. I walked a little taller, a little happier, a little stronger, a little longer, all the while telling Mrs. Crooks that she had been served!

Mrs. Crooks and her rowdy kids are in constant pursuit. Chaos and fear are their go-to weapons. They use it to create clutter, clogging up your pathways of faith-filled actions with fear-filled calamity. If I would have just paused, even if just for a minute to gather myself, breathe, and *pray*, I would have tapped into the power that was already inside of me.

My mother would always tell me to put it in the "God Box," an imaginary or real box to place your worries, fears, and challenges, because nothing is too big for God. But I relied on my flesh and took out the wrong weapons—weapons that caused me to wreak havoc on my emotional health.

Through worry, I spoke death. Through fear, I spoke defeat. I was so busy caught up in their game that I forgot my superpowers. I started claiming something that was unconfirmed. Do you get this? By signing up to get notifications about an illness that didn't exist in my body, I waved the white flag of surrender when I should have been raising my hands to the Heavenly Father claiming the victory. Victory that no matter what the results were, I was going to face it with the same strength and resiliency with which I faced every other situation that showed up in my life.

My initial response to Dr. Lemley's call reporting the worrisome lab results wasn't prayer or stillness, but an overwhelming bout of fear and a "why me?" attitude. I didn't handle this journey the right way. This doesn't mean that when faced with life's challenges, we must put up a heroic or invincible front. We're human, and when life throws tomatoes at us, they do splatter and create a mess. Acknowledge it, but don't ever give up your power.

In *Super Genes*, Chopra and Tanzi speak to revolutionizing our approach to health down to the cellular level. Their hope is to raise the bar on the power we must employ to change our gene activity. They go on to say, "Every cell is eavesdropping on what you think, say, and do."

This one sentence made me think of biblical principles and the power we must speak over our lives and the lives of others. Life and death are in the power of the tongue. I realized I was speaking death. Down to the deepest part of my makeup, I told my cells that they were defective. I added the burden of yet another condition to battle. An unnecessary burden. The stress and worry I imposed for more than two months sent the wrong messages. I chose to allow my cells to eavesdrop on a conversation I really didn't want them to hear, let alone process as truth. Mrs. Crooks got me! She robbed me of peace. I not only backed off on the eviction notices, I gave her a few free nights in the penthouse.

I guarantee you there will be a next time, but I will be ready when that times comes. I will be ready. I will arm myself with the spiritual weapons needed to be victorious. I will not succumb to fear. I will approach it the Philippians 4:6 way, "Do not be anxious about anything, but in everything, by prayer and petition, with thanksgiving, present your requests to God."

Lesson 9

Make Every Moment Count

WHEN MY MOM, KARIMA, WAS IN HER THIRTIES, SHE STARTED complaining of symptoms that mirrored diabetes. She was subsequently diagnosed with Type I—insulin dependent—diabetes.

As a teenager, hearing the word "diabetes" meant little to my siblings and me. My mom looked great, she continued to walk everywhere, and her vibrant nature never waned. That's the tricky and cruel thing about diabetes' vengeance. Its destructive path can go unnoticed for quite some time until the damage manifests itself in the way of kidney disease, tingling in your toes and hands, eye problems, and issues with blood flow through your organs and extremities. My mom kept it moving and so did diabetes. Diabetes did what it does best by slowly destroying the rooms of my mother's temple.

"I'm oxidizing." That was a statement that could only come from my mom. I mean, who would use the word "oxidizing" to describe what was happening to their body? "Oxidizing" was not a word I wanted to hear come out of my mother's mouth, especially since I didn't need Webster's Dictionary to tell me what she meant.

Oxidation is the interaction of oxygen molecules with the substances they touch. Oxidation in the body is also known as aging. To slow the process of oxidation, you need to be healthy and to boost your immunity with antioxidants. My mother had such a command of the English language that carrying Webster in your pocket wasn't such a bad idea. Engaging in conversation with my mom was sure to be a lyrical experience. She was a poet, orator, teacher, and radio personality all in one petite package.

My mom's declaration of her body oxidizing symbolized that her decreased immunity and fragile state of illness had gotten to the point of no return. My mom knew the state of her health. She was dying, and had been over the course of years, but today's choice of words was to let me know that her time was soon to come.

I really wasn't in the mood to hear this. Over the past few years, my mom did her best to prepare her girls for this time. I wasn't ready! I wanted to revert to my mom's cheerful, pumped-up coaching calls that got my day started on the right foot. I craved this time with my mom. No matter what I was facing, my mom made me feel that my victory was already won and no one, not a single soul, had the power to take anything away from me.

My mom didn't believe in wallowing in defeat. Her motto was, "Let forward and upward always be your motion." Even if she believed the situation was dire, my mom would never allow a spirit of defeat to overcome you. She was the consummate mentor, coach, and inspirer. My mom made it clear that she knew the end was near. Her wish was that I faced this moment with strength and courage. That was a tall order for me.

In many ways, I was still Sunshine, hanging out the window and begging her to take me to the co-op. She knew that adjusting to life without her would be difficult. Together, we were both journeying through some of life's most heartbreaking tragedies. Sharing a bond of losing our sons is a commonality we wish we didn't have, yet it was the one that fueled us to feed each other hope.

My mom's primary goal over the past few years was to make sure her girls were going to be okay. She was insistent on her approach to prepare, or more like threaten, our husbands to take good care of us, love us through the pain, and carry us when standing on our own was unbearable. My mom also spent a lot of time making sure my sister and I would grow even closer, and be there for each other and hold our family up in her absence. To say she was the matriarch is an understatement. She was both light and life. A fierce protector. From her great-grandchildren to her great aunts and uncles, everyone wanted more of my mom's life.

Having just returned from a visit with my mom during a trip to Philadelphia for the Pennsylvania Conference for Women, I certainly didn't want to think that would be my last time in my mom's presence. The conference took place at the best time of the year. I would get to celebrate my birthday with my mom and enjoy a great conference that brought together inspiring women on a mission.

In retrospect, there were signs, glaring signs, that my mom was preparing for her transition. Just a month prior to the conference, my mom wanted to host one of our family dinners at my sister's home. When family members began to cancel and other life happenings got in the way, she still wanted to move forward with dinner. When I look back at the pictures taken during our September gathering, it was clear that my mom was taking it all in. A deep expression of reflection on her face appeared on every photo. It was as if she was capturing every moment.

After the conference, it was time to make my way back to Pittsburgh. Before pulling off, I looked up at the bedroom that became my mom's final living space in my sister's home. As if on cue, her petite silhouette appeared in the window. Even in the darkness of the early morning, I could still see the clear expression on her face. It was a look of longing for just a little more time. Not just the time between my monthly trips back home, but more time on Earth, more time in a healthier state of being, more time experiencing life in all its beauty and pain. Just more time.

Mom stood in the window, waving goodbye, sending kisses, and smiling a smile that said more than any words could express. Yes, I could feel the difference in this morning's goodbye. It was as if we were both in a trance, a futile attempt to hold onto something deeper than goodbye. Our eyes locked and spoke a history of love, struggle, and triumph that distance on this plane of consciousness or the next would never sever. That was October 6, 2012.

"Mom, I really don't want to hear that, besides, who calls up their daughter first thing in the morning telling her, 'I'm oxidizing'? Anyway, Dr. Ntoso told us a few years ago that your medical conditions and prognosis was bad and getting out of 2009 alive would be a miracle. Well, I guess miracles still do happen because it's been three years and you're still here. There's no way you're leaving me now. You've conquered worse and I'm simply not ready, nor will I ever be ready to journey this life without you."

We didn't take Dr. Ntoso's statement for granted. As a nurse, mother, and sister who has experienced unpredictable loss, I choose to wring the life out of life. If we all treated each moment as if it were truly our last, I believe life would be experienced at a much higher level. I know intimately the limitations of making statements around how much time someone has to live, and I know that physicians don't take these declarations lightly. What Dr. Ntoso was doing was trying to prepare us for the worse-case scenario based on his experience practicing medicine. So, over the three years prior, my mom soaked up life. We created memories and moments that would be forever etched in our hearts and minds.

On October 8, 2012, my mom spent the day driving in her Jeep, blasting music, and dropping greeting cards in the mailbox. She was an avid card sender. My mom made sure everyone knew they were being thought of. The cards came unexpectedly, not just on birthdays or special occasions, they were sent with love *just because.* That evening was spent having dinner with Samira, my brother-in-law, Terry, and my niece, Amira. My mom even spent a few minutes on the treadmill. She had a good day.

There's a paralyzing and fear-stricken anxiety that overcomes me when the phone rings in the middle of the night. One too many times, midnight calls have greeted me with tragedy and conditioned me to expect the worst. My initial reaction to the ringing phone was to ignore it, as if it were merely a figment of my imagination, or even better, someone calling the wrong number. I was tired of being held hostage to bad news via a phone call. Why else would someone call at this hour? Who would be up at this time of the morning bearing good news?

Call it courage or learning how to stand up and face life head on, but I knew I had to pick it up. It was Samira, and based on the noise I heard in the background, this was not a joy call. I don't know exactly when I zoned out. I tried my best to pull myself together, put on my nurse hat, and assist my sister. But the sound, the rhythmic grunts coming from my mom, terrified me.

The grunts played like horrible background music that I couldn't tune out. "Is that mom?" I asked.

We sometimes ask questions that we know the answers to, but we hold on to some outrageous notion that even when we're 100 percent right, we grasp at the desire to be proven wrong.

"Yes, that's Mom," my sister said.

"She can't talk?" I asked.

"No," Samira replied. She tried her best to explain what she was witnessing.

I tried to put my nurse hat on as calmly as I could, but I was so focused on the grunting sound coming from my mom. "What happened?" I asked.

Samira went on to explain that her husband, Terry, woke up in the middle of the night to use the bathroom and heard a noise coming from my mom's room. My sister ran into the room to find her on the floor, still connected to her peritoneal dialysis machine and making grunting sounds. Although my mom couldn't speak, she seemed to understand my sister's questions and nodded or grunted appropriately in response.

It was a known fact that my mom wasn't too fond of Western medicine. She often referred to physicians as Dr. Frankenstein and one, as the Alien.

Over the course of my mom's illness, Samira and I had become connected to her physicians and dialysis team. They were like extended family. We were blessed by the way they cared for my mom. We knew my mom was a handful, and her health care providers quickly found out the same.

Samira and I were given strict instructions on my mom's end-of-life wishes. She was clear that she would be the one to convince us that ghosts exist if we kept her hooked up to life-saving, "frankensteinish" machines. "No machines or I'll haunt you," my mom said. When Samira asked my mom if she wanted to go to the hospital, and my mom's grunt and head nod said yes, I knew it was bad.

Hate is a strong word, but that was the only feeling I could convey toward diabetes. This disease was wreaking havoc on my family. Me, my mom, Samira, and my mom's sister, Aunt Yakini, were all being attacked by diabetes. It had already killed my mom's father when she was only eight years old.

I watched diabetes pick my mom apart. Fighting back with an emotion of hate isn't the answer to killing diabetes, but in that moment, it was the only response to the pain. A free-spirit and lover of life, my mom lost her freedom to diabetes' greedy clutch. Blindness, heart disease, kidney disease, and now this: no ability to speak, just grunts.

Samira and I were a team. We helped each other on this dark and heavy morning, 300 miles apart, trying desperately to get my mom the help she needed to live. Samira followed the ambulance while I rushed off the phone to find a flight that would get me home.

I pleaded in prayer for God to have mercy on my mom's life. *I'm not ready! I need her,* I thought. The little girl that slept with her mom until she was a teen needed her. The same little girl that would run to keep up with her needed her. I was crying out for just a little more time. Losing my son was enough! No more loss. Please. My mom's efforts to prepare us for what could be our last moment with her weren't going so well.

I'm convinced that loss, whether you have time to prepare or it's unexpected, still hurts like hell. I was set up to not accept death from my very first experience watching the snake eat breakfast in Ms. Rhoda's first grade class. As sweet as Ms. Rhoda was in trying her best to explain the circle of life, I simply wasn't ready to receive that lesson. From that moment on, two things became my enemies: snakes and death! And today, I was no closer to acceptance.

My mom was only fifty-seven years old. A few years before her death, she would point out that she had already surpassed the age when her mother died at forty-one. That was always painful to hear. In my mind, neither my mom nor my grandmother experienced growing old.

"I want to live," my mom said during a conversation. She burst into tears and said, "I want my eyesight. I want my kidneys to function, and I want to walk fast again." Now she couldn't even talk.

After multiple flight delays, I made it to Philadelphia. I remember begging the attendant at the flight gate to help me. I knew she had no control, but I was so desperate to find a way to be at my mom's side. My sister asked the doctor to withhold the severity of my mom's condition, but I knew. Just like it felt like eternity getting to Philadelphia after my son's death, the flight to get to my mom was the same feeling.

After my flight landed, I was greeted with a heavy sadness that spread across my Abi and youngest sister Naeemah's faces. We rushed to the hospital as quick as we could. I was directed to my mom's room in the ER. My body went limp when I saw my mom connected to life support. I dropped. No, this can't be the end. The ER doctor asked if we knew my mom's end of life wishes.

Samira and I looked at one another silently, sharing a promise that we didn't want to honor. My mom was explicitly clear that by no means would she want to be kept on life support. Yes, we knew, but we wanted to hold on just a little while longer. I wanted to ask if they had any more tubes they could hook her up to. Yes, we knew. My mom knew too. She knew her girls were not strong enough to let go.

The doctor said he would give us time to say goodbye before removing the "frankensteinish" machine that kept my mom alive. The sounds that indicated proof of life started to slow down.

As I lay in the hospital bed with my mom, the same way I laid in the bed with her as a child, my sister later told me she prayed I would make it to the hospital in time. She asked my mom in her final state of transition to hold on just a little while longer. My sister knew hours before I arrived there was no coming back from this. My mom had suffered a massive hemorrhagic stroke. They had no intervention, no cure.

I turned to look up at the machine that captured her heartbeat and other vital signs. My mom was taking it out of our hands. She knew, God knew, and the decision was made for us.

October 9, 2012, my mom died in our arms. We whispered sweet words in her ears. Within minutes of my arrival, my mom transitioned into peace. And now we had to figure out how we were going to do what my mom always taught us: keep it moving!

Lesson 10

The Voice Within

THERE WERE DISTINCT PEARLS OF WISDOM MY MOM PASSED down that have served me well into adulthood. She instilled in me a warrior spirit that helped me to thrive and not just survive when faced with life's most horrific tragedies.

One Mommy Mantra that I learned at an early age was "to struggle is to win." My mom didn't believe in giving up. No matter how much she felt the weight of the world pressing down on her 4'11, one hundred-pound frame, nothing would keep her down.

I can hear my mom saying, "When you fall down, you better get back up." It was amazing how her larger-than-life personality was wrapped up in this petite package. There was never a need to interpret what my mom meant when she spoke. You didn't have to like her delivery; you got the message.

My mom's presence was felt in every environment she stepped in, and as a radio personality, poet, teacher, and author, she used both the English and French languages—if you know what I mean—in an unapologetic way. Her uniqueness was as free as the wild horses running across the beaches of Assateague Island. These horses are often described as being tough, beautiful, and wild. Those same characteristics paint a story about my mom's life. Just like the wild horses of Assateague have learned to survive the brutality of a harsh environment, so did she.

On a recent trip to Arizona to visit my bonus children, we stopped at a dude ranch to enjoy horseback riding. To say my horseback riding skills were rusty is an understatement, especially since it's been twenty-five years since I rode a horse. I was both nervous and excited about this adventure. I trained and cared for horses along with other farm animals while attending WB Saul High School of Agricultural Science. I loved that experience in high school, but it also left me with a scar.

Horses are just as temperamental as people. If fear was in the air, they used it to their full advantage. I've been kicked, thrown off, and in a face-to-face standoff. The horses surely won all their battles with me. I wanted to escape the memories of the not-so-good time with horses to enjoy the moment.

We wanted to have a full experience during our trip. My sister-in-law, Jennifer, being the ever-wonderful planner, found a great horseback riding deal on one of her Groupon searches. In just one day, we went from wintry, city weather to a warm, sunny desert.

A cloud of dust enveloped our car as we drove down the dirt road to the dude ranch. The ranch looked like it was plucked straight out of one of those old cowboy flicks. The ones that always seem to occupy my husband's Saturday mornings. The guy leading us on our Wild West adventure had us pegged. I watched how he surveyed the group and subtly assigned the horses as if he could smell the fear dripping from the smiles plastered on our faces. I was secretly praying that he pegged me for a wimp. I didn't mind getting the horse that was on his way to horsey heaven. Slow and safe was my motto for the journey. My only goal was to begin and finish this journey with all body parts intact.

Jennifer ended up with the horse with one foot in horsey heaven. After witnessing how darn slow it was, I was quite satisfied with the four-legged friend chosen for me.

I found out some interesting things on our western trail adventure. My husband had an inner cowboy that I had no clue about. He ended up with the worst behaving horse I've ever seen. This horse was truly the problem child. If there was a diagnosis of attention deficit for horses, he surely had it. I was terrified of him. He didn't listen, purposely tried to throw my husband off, and was just downright rude. He was surely not on board with the fact we paid for this experience and wanted to leave alive.

I watched in pure amazement at how my husband handled him. There was zero fear, and, quite frankly, my husband did a great job of showing this horse who was in charge. The other horses just seemed to follow the routine. There was a knowing among the horses that this was their life. These trails were familiar territory. They waited for their daily work of riding visitors from all over the country hyped up about a western adventure. Day in, day out.

After about an hour riding along the trail, something unexpected happened. Out of the desert bushes, several unbridled wild horses appeared. Their stature was different than the horses we were riding. They stood with a visible strength; heads held high, chest pronounced as if to say to our horses, "What in the world are you guys doing? What's all that crap on you, and what are those things riding on your backs?"

They just stood and stared as we rode by. I stayed back for as long as I could just to take them in. They reminded me of my mom. They looked at me as if my mom sent them to ask me similar questions: "What are you doing with your life? Why are you carrying all that crap?"

I was grateful for the signs, even if they were all made up in my mind. I was making a choice to not walk through life with blinders, neither bridled nor saddled down. I was noticing that I wasn't going to be rescued. Although my husband was living out his dream to be a cowboy that would save the day, watching the free, unbridled horses was a message that I had to be the one to rescue my damn self. I needed to consider what I chose to continue carrying through life: the weight of pain, grief, disappointment, and fear. I had to answer the question about what I was doing and how long was I going to stay there.

That dude ranch experience and the crossing of the wild horses made me realize the freedom I had. I could choose to pack the heavy baggage, day in or day out, or I could make a different choice and choose a lighter load.

There's a voice within guiding us in the right direction. Sometimes, we just need to be still enough to listen, and then rise with a strong conviction and a response that brings forth the light.

Part III

Why You Were Born

Atiya's Living Room

FOR LASTING CHANGE TO OCCUR IN OUR LIVES, WE MUST take deliberate steps to internalize the experiences we're meant to learn from. One of my most profound experiences happened during Oprah's The Life You Want weekend tour.

The Verizon Center in Washington, DC was the venue where more than 10,000 people gathered to begin the work of creating the life they dreamed of. During one of the breaks, I patiently stood in the restroom line hoping that it wouldn't take a lifetime to get through it. Listening to the women sharing their renewed hope and excitement helped me to deal with my impending bladder rupture. By no means is holding your bladder a practice I'd endorse, but the experience in the conference was one you didn't want to risk missing a second of. I tried my best not to look awkward as I shifted positions to hold on just a little bit longer.

During the chatter, a fellow Oprahite walked by me with that, *I know you* look on her face. She stopped after walking a few feet from the restroom line, turned around and said, "I'm sorry but you look very familiar. Tracy Lynn, right?"

I shook my head and replied, "No."

"But you look awfully familiar," said the woman.

Our conversation felt more like a tennis match with the back and forth banter. We couldn't shake it off, so we verbally went through our checklist starting with our names, place of birth, current residence, job, and social security numbers—well, we didn't go that far, but it felt like an eternity before we figured it out. Ah-ha! It was when she shared she was living in York, Pennsylvania that it hit me.

I responded, "I host the Fun, Fit & Fabulous women's health conference in Hershey, Pennsylvania, which isn't too far from York." Bingo! So, in Washington, DC, amid more than 10,000 people, we met again.

The woman replied, "That's it! I was in your living room two weeks ago."

The living room this woman referred to wasn't my actual living room. The living room she sat in was filled with more than 200 of my "girlfriends." This special living room was a workshop I facilitated at the twelfth annual Fun, Fit & Fabulous Women's Health Conference. I didn't know until the last minute that I was to facilitate a session. When I saw my name on the agenda, I asked my team member, "Am I conducting a workshop?"

She replied, "Yes."

I responded, "Well, what do you want me to do in this workshop?"

My coworker said, "Just do you." Enough said!

I gathered the keynote speaker and three other workshop presenters into a huddle, and I said, "Follow my lead. We are going to help these women remove some of those hats they wear everyday which prevent them from depositing into their own lives." I wanted to create a safe environment where these women could freely express their feelings around the roles they assume every day and the roles they dreamed of assuming to truly live a fun, fit, and fabulous life.

I titled my session, "Atiya's Living Room." The only hat that each woman was asked to wear was a crown. The only person I wanted them to save was themselves. My mom always told me, "self-preservation is not selfishness, but self-love, and that is where it all begins." The three other magnificent speakers shared insight and encouragement, which helped each woman design a plan that put them at the top of their to-do list.

The woman I met in the restroom line happened to be one of the women sitting in my "living room" at the conference. The miracle of her appearing right in front of me was a reminder that the life I was creating, the journey I was on, is much bigger than me. Her presence ushered me even further on the path of being a living, breathing example of the *why* behind the journey.

The excitement of us finally figuring out how our paths crossed died down, and what was left was a warm smile and a thoughtful but silent stare into each other's eyes. "You are right where you were meant to be."

Her response broke our daze. She reflected on what she experienced in *Atiya's Living Room*. She recalled the conviction and calling to help women create a life that didn't place their needs at the bottom of the to-do list. She thanked me for that experience, and I thanked her for being present.

On this weekend, I and 9,999 others were getting about the business of designing the rest of our lives, the best of our lives. Showing up didn't symbolize that we had it all together, or that our plans were foolproof. Showing up meant we were not going to waste another moment wishing for what our lives would have been like if we put fire under the life we really wanted. That experience with Oprah, the spiritual trailblazers she brought along, and that woman who sat in Atiya's Living Room, were all my miracle reminders of the life I wanted. Now how could I continue walking through life ignoring that?

I would have denied myself the beauty in these life encounters if I didn't muster up enough faith, love, and courage to save my own. After losing my son, I felt lost and purposeless. When Oprah shared her journey with us, she often talked about having faith. And not just any kind of faith, but sunrise faith.

She described it as a kind of faith that no matter how difficult life becomes, you believe the sun will still rise. I don't take it for granted that I'm still here bearing witness to sunrises and sunsets. The past has been filled with more pain and more losses than I can count. But I can't acknowledge the pain without sharing the beautiful bursts of blessings.

I did more than just hold on and merely survive. I learned how to breathe again, smile again, and live again. I learned that living to your highest calling is the most important gift you can give to honor your loved ones, those who are no longer here to witness the sunrise and sunset.

If You Could Save One Person

EACH OF US HAS A RESPONSIBILITY TO HONOR THE CALLING on our lives. It's important not to get your calling confused with fame or fortune. The inspiration for writing this book was stalled because I was more focused on the grand scale of things instead of the one life I could touch.

There's power in numbers, but don't let that determine whether you hold back important information about your journey that can help someone else. I was stuck for a long time. Fear kept rearing its ugly, obnoxious head every time I got close to the finish line. Thoughts about what others would think consumed me. Mom called this voice "The Whisperer." In my head, I kept hearing, *everyone has a story; why is yours worth telling?*

The Whisperer preyed on my self-inflicted, defeatist attitude. *Do you really want them to know that?* She was adept at knowing what pain points to push, the ones that send you into an abyss of questions designed to keep you spiraling in doubt. I couldn't stand her—or me, since I'm being honest. When I extended an invitation for her to have a voice at *my* table, I gave up way too much control. And I was sick of living like that.

But I didn't stop there because I said she could bring a friend, so procrastination showed up. It hit me just how much control I relinquished when Rob Wilson, Financial Expert and Dream Catcher—my name for him—asked me one question: "What are you currently struggling with?"

"My book," I replied. "I can't finish it unless I make it so important that nothing will get in the way."

I gave Rob all the sexy excuses The Whisperer made me believe. I had way too much on my plate, with work, family, renovating an historic property, moving, hosting and planning shows, and helping my family. The list became a never-ending saga as to why I couldn't buckle down and get it done. Did I mention *fear*? Yeah, that no-good rat showed up too.

I envisioned Rob reading my list of excuses, shaking his head, and saying, "Haven't I heard all this before?" I was singing the same tired tune many of us sing when we're afraid. I found myself encouraging others to ditch The Whisperer and procrastination, but I had a hard time *internalizing* the same message.

Rob's response was an indication he wasn't buying the crap I was trying to sell. If I really wanted to help someone else, that woman, that girl who was struggling to move forward, the person who can't fathom the possibility of moving on and going from merely surviving to thriving, then I would have finished my book yesterday. That's what Rob said. His words, written in a nice, but get-yo-stuff-together kind of way, revealed that Someday Syndrome had gotten the best of me.

Atiya,

Thanks for sharing that with me. In my experience, there are a few major reasons why people get stuck: Their WHY isn't clear enough or strong enough and/or they don't believe that whatever they have been putting off will actually get the results that they desire for them. So, perhaps you should focus on your __why__? Maybe there is one individual life that you should focus on. When you write, act as if you are writing to her and use that as your inspiration. If you __truly__ want to enlighten, encourage and empower, it is your duty to get this information out into the world. If you could save one person's life, just one, would you want to not have done it because you were too busy?

Or, you may not strongly feel as though your book will get the results that you desire. You might be wondering if you will really be able to save a life with your writing. I know you can get over this. Because, in my opinion, if you could be absolutely 100% certain that your book would save some-one's life, you would have it done yesterday. Don't second guess yourself. We all have fears that we are inadequate in one way or another. If you take the focus away from yourself and make it about "her," you'll find that it will be much easier for you to get the words out.

Now, I know that what Rob did for me is something that he does for countless others. It's his special gift to not only help you ignite your dreams, but to make sure that you're doing it in a financially sound way. For the sake of my journey, I'd like to believe Rob is a part of the God network, keeping people like me from falling so far and so deep that you miss your purpose.

Rob's words were the antidote against The Whisperer's taunts of inadequacy and fear. He was placed in my life for such a time as this. Rob's gentle, but bam-in-your-face nudge, reminded me of why I was still breathing, and why I believed, amid the pain, that my life was worth saving.

When I count my blessings, I count the many people who have not let me give up on life. These individuals are on assignment, carrying out duties that help others to not sleepwalk through life. I kept Rob's words in my purse, folded up on a piece of paper. Every time I felt the urge to throw in the towel, I would be reminded that my story wasn't for me alone.

Not for You Alone

IT WAS THE 2008 FUN, FIT & FABULOUS WOMEN'S HEALTH Conference. Just two weeks after marrying Tim in Riviera Maya, Mexico. I was on a high. Tim was in the back serving as my assistant, and I was in the front sharing my story.

After the session, I received a profound request, one that up until then I hadn't even considered. A young woman came up to the front of the room, with tears streaming down her face. We stood face to face, holding hands.

"I want more of this. Do you have a book?" she asked.

I tilted my head, smiled, and responded with what I know was a quizzical look. "More?" I replied.

"Yes, a book," she said again. Tears continued to stream down her face while we stood there holding hands.

I made a promise to her that day. A promise to give her more. More to that woman, that person, who yearned for more hope, more courage, more love, and more strength to live an incredible life dancing in the sun and strutting through the storm. I wanted so much to share the overwhelming power we have to change our *story*.

My encounter with that woman changed my life. She gave me an assignment. An assignment that put me on a path that was so much bigger than the moment we shared. I believe, like Rob, this young woman was also a part of the God network, sent as a messenger. Like many of us, she wanted to discover the power of the human spirit to go on to live a joy-filled life, one that wasn't based on the dream of a pain-free existence.

We often find ourselves wishing for just that: pain-free. But that promise wasn't given to us. There is strength, peace, and joy that is resurrected out of the pit of darkness. It causes us to rise through the pain and move forward and upward like nobody's business. That young woman helped me in ways she may never know—or maybe she does!

My husband and I left the conference the next day, and discovered a nice, quaint restaurant to enjoy brunch and write the outline to the book you're reading now. I couldn't believe I was going to do this, but then I thought, *why not*? It's my story and who better to tell it than me. If this book could help facilitate the healing we all have a right to experience, then I didn't have any time to waste.

Life has taught me some important lessons. One, I'm not on a list. I'm not being punished. The only promise God made was that I would not travel the heartache road alone. Life taught me to capture the moments, create memories, and cherish people and experiences, not things. Love and love again; forgive, and keep on forgiving.

Life has taught me that the piercings from the pain may never go away, but God's grace is indeed sufficient. His grace extends through the love and kindness of others. My journey is clearly not a fairytale, but it is a faith tale. I know some parts are heavy—very heavy. In all its beauty and pain, it's still my story. It's my declaration that this journey isn't mine for safe keeping. And neither is yours. It's one to be shared.

For when that woman—or man—walks up to you with tears streaming down their face, asking you for more, you can look them straight in their eyes and know in that very moment, your journey is not for you alone. Our connectedness to one another is part of our prescription for a life worth saving. It's showing up every day even when you want to hide under the covers.

Rob said that if I believed that my story could help just one person, I would have written it yesterday. So, when I'm caught up in those moments—struggling, falling, and getting up—something more powerful than me stirs in my soul and whispers, *Someone, somewhere, needs to know their life is worth saving!*

I hope that someone is you!

Epilogue

IT HAS BEEN LONG JOURNEY TO GET THIS BOOK INTO THE world. A lot has transpired since I started focusing on the editing process of this book two years ago. I've learned acceptance brings peace and everything serves a purpose, even the so-called delays in life.

We relocated to Jacksonville, Florida after Tim received an incredible opportunity to serve in a new role. I obtained a PhD in Community Engagement and now they call me Dr. A. In the midst of these major life transitions, saving my life has been a hard and cyclical process. I continue to bear witness to the power of connectedness. My beloved creatures continued to demonstrate that healing comes in various forms.

Dory stayed alongside me and Nemo for as long as she could. The first year in Florida I noticed her stride getting a little slower. She bumped into things often and it would scare the life out of me watching her run down my long apartment hallway knowing she would come so close to colliding into the wall. When the violent seizures started, I knew her time with us was coming to an end. The thought of losing my sweet Dory tore me up inside. The new veterinarian was aware of our story and helped sustain her life as long as possible. At some point it was pure selfishness trying to keep her on this side of consciousness. Just two days before Tim's birthday in 2018, after a sustained and violent seizure that wouldn't end, we found ourselves at the emergency hospital. And just like Buddy, I held onto Dory and cried into her white ball of fur when the veterinarian informed me it was time to let her go. This time Tim didn't protest me holding her while the medications lulled her into a permanent sleep. He just held onto Nemo, who I was hoping was unaware of what was happening to his partner. As Dory looked at me with her big, droopy eyes I told her just how much she rescued me and loved me back to life. At fourteen years old I wanted her to be around a little longer. My heart felt just enough peace knowing her latter years were certainly greater. I guess you could say we loved each other back to life. As she took her last breath I assured her and Tim and Nemo that I would *just keep swimming*.

Swimming is just what I did and my family did too. My bonus son blessed us with two granddaughters. My goddaughter who I helped bring into the world as her nurse and had the pleasure of co-raising is now a college freshman. My daughter is a biomolecular scientist working on research at UC San Diego and my youngest son has started his own clothing line. Tim is still Tim. Loving and worrying about his wife. I've asked for a kayak, a paddleboard, and to experience indoor skydiving and just like with the marathon experience, his answer remains NO. It's okay, for I know his protective nature only comes from a deep concern and love for his wife's wellbeing. I've maintained a healthy weight, gained twenty pounds during my PhD journey and lost it again. My family continues to grow stronger, together. Living in Florida hasn't prevented me from spending quality time, traveling, and capturing moments with my lifelines.

There's healing power in being socially connected and the way I was designed is to fill up with the fuel of family, including my four siblings, friends, and experiences. I'm settling into a healthy stride with a few health scares but always bounced back. I've added coping mechanisms that help me survive the tsunami of grief that is still ever present. The thorns I carry continue to pierce my side; I've just learned to manage them with the beautiful roses they produce. I'm using my journey to the highest level. My spirit of transparency has touched the lives of others. My life is an open book and I'm perfectly okay with that. The assignment God has given me is more important than what others may think, say, or do. I'm reminded that what people think of me is none of my business but what God thinks of me dictates my movement. I'm leveraging my experiences to help women lead their lives with wellbeing and help communities restore, heal, and build, all while pursuing the fun things that bring my life joy. I relocated my father to Florida to receive treatment for a rare and life-threatening disease. Having my father, my Abi with us has brought more joy, more love, more responsibility into our lives. My Abi has shared deeply personal accounts of my creation and the true meaning of my name. Through this experience with him I have received confirmation that my life is unfolding in a manner that honors my existence and charges me with the responsibility to help others honor theirs.

Acknowledgments

LIFE HAS TAUGHT ME THAT NOTHING IS MORE IMPORTANT than the people who make life worth living. I am most grateful to the two human beings responsible for bringing me on the planet. My mom, who taught me what it meant to be a warrior and to fight for my life. Her free spirit has inspired me to break the rules and do what brings my heart the most joy. My dad, Abi, has and will always be my biggest supporter. He helped me navigate the rough waters of life and not spend a lifetime crying over spilled milk.

My family and friends, thank you for showing me what it truly means to love unconditionally. Your incredible support and guidance have helped me navigate life's rough terrain. You celebrated with me in victory and loved me through the difficult parts of my journey. And for that, I'm grateful!

There are parts of my journey that were so rough that I wanted out. Three human beings watched their mother travel through the worst and best of times. They are my breath! Keemy, you have given me a meaning worth living for. I wish you were here to see your mom all grown up. Cierra, you were a blessing from the first time I laid eyes on you. Thanks for always believing in your mom and showing me what brave looks like. Diante, a true momma's boy, I am so proud of the man you're becoming. You're my champion, encouraging me to reach for the stars. And that's exactly what I want for you.

To my Highmark family, I don't know if you know just how big of a role you played in my life, but choosing this company helped saved me.

Dr. Hanlon, aka Dr. H., it's all your fault! Thank you for starting this process of writing. It has become a very important part of my healing journey.

With the exception of my dissertation, I have never written anything this extensive in my life! Phyllis, Tim, and Samira, thank you for all the helpful feedback and editing.

Tieffa and Elizabeth, my heart is full! Your incredible support as my editor and encourager has allowed me to bring my truth into the world. I am eternally grateful!

Karen, I truly believe everyone deserves someone like you in their lives. Your gifts will make a way for you! I thank you for using your unmatched talent as my creative director and knowing me so well that you're able to capture the essence of every experience and turn them into masterpieces. Your gentle nudge, your love, and your friendship fuel my spirit. I am closer than I think!

Tim and I have such a beautiful, blended family. My heart is full because of your presence. Jason, Lauren, Cierra, Diante, Juliet,Our granddaughters Ava and Aria, and our goddaughter Lexi. Thank you! You make life worth living!

Tim, you represent so much in my life. We love hard and battle hard but love always wins! You're my hubby, my friend, my prayer partner, my love, and the man who reads his wife bedtime stories. It doesn't get much better than that. Thank you for riding the waves of our never-dull life. We ended up exactly where we were meant to be: together.

Hakeem, my "Keemy," thank you for showing me through your life the greatest gifts of love and forgiveness. I will honor your existence by honoring mine. Love and light son!